A COMPREHENSIVE BOOK OF OBJECTIVE STRUCTURED CLINICAL EXAMINATION (OSCE) IN GENERAL MEDICINE

Authors:

Dr. Sunil Kumar

Dr. Sourya Acharya

Co Authors:

Dhruv Talwar, Rinkle Gemnani

Department of Medicine, Jawaharlal Nehru Medical College,
Datta Meghe Institute of higher education and research (Deemed to be University),
Wardha, Maharashtra, India. 442001

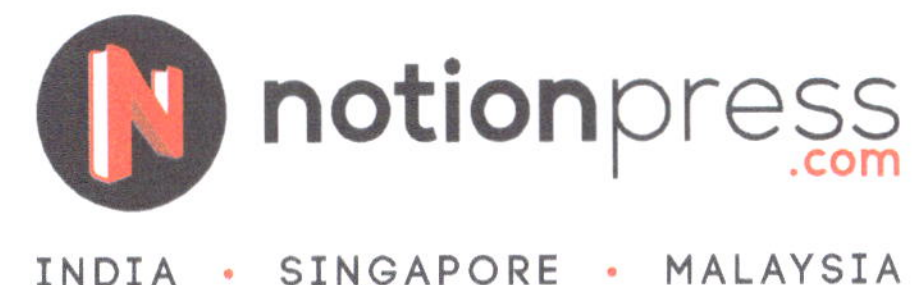

ISBN 979-8-89363-267-5

Dedicated to

All Our Students

Index

About the Authors

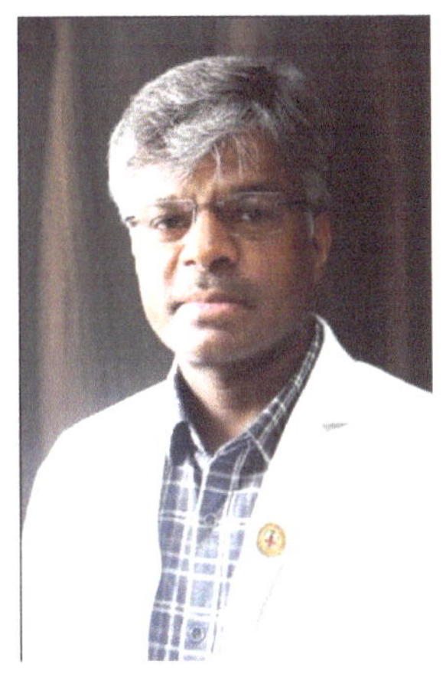

Dr Sunil Kumar (MBBS, MD, PhD): The lead author has authored various book chapters in international books, original research articles on topic ranging from general medicine, geriatric medicine, and critical care in various international journals with high impact factor. The author has teaching experience of more than 20 years in medical college with undergraduate, post-graduate, doctoral and fellowship courses. He has also completed a Basic and advanced course in medical education technology and has published a paper related to medical education. With his keen interest in research and teaching experience, he has done justice to the requirement of a book, which caters to the curriculum needs of undergraduate as well as post-graduate students in General Medicine.

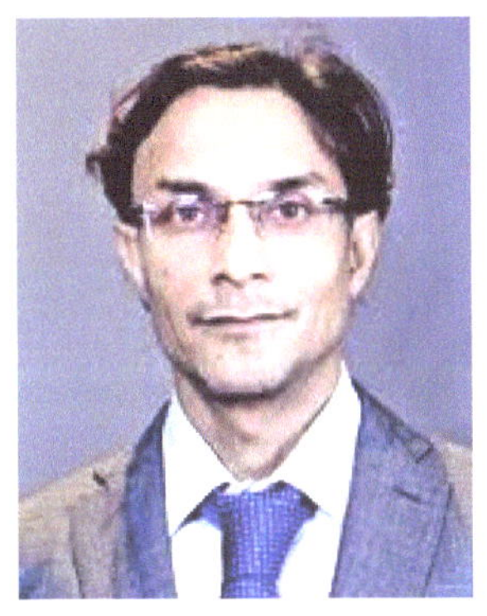

Dr. Sourya Acharya [MBBS, DNB, PhD (Internal Medicine)]: He is a Professor and Head, Dept. of Medicine, Jawaharlal Nehru Medical College. Wardha, Maharashtra. He is a clinician, academician and researcher. He has 20 years of teaching experience; is a Reviewer of reputed Journals. He is also a Life member API IMA Member American college of Physicians, has Fellowship in Critical care Medicine, APPOLLO Hyderabad, IMA recognized clinical instructor in Clinical cardiology, Clinical Diabetes, Rheumatology. He has More than 200 publications in various national and International indexed medical journals. He has Done Basic and Advanced Course in Medical Education and Technology, DMIMSDU Nodal Center. He is recipient of BAPIO Award for Excellence in Teaching and Mentoring.

Corresponding author:

Sunil Kumar MD, PhD
Professor
Department of Medicine
JawaharLal Nehru Medical College, Datta Meghe Institute of higher education and research (Deemed to be University), Wardha, Maharashtra, India. 442001
9850393787
Email – sunilkumarmed@gmail.com

Contributors

- Dr. AK Wanjari
- Dr.Shilpa Bawankule
- Dr Keyur Saboo
- Dr Nikhil Pantbalekundri
- Dr Vinit Deolikar
- Dr Venkat Reddy
- Dr Abhinav Kadam
- Dr Kashish Khurana
- Dr Varun Daiya
- Dr SaketToshniwal
- Dr Nitish Batra
- Dr Rucha Sawant
- Dr Harshita Reddy
- Dr Palash Kotak
- Dr Pranav Chaudhary
- Dr Sarang Raut
- Dr Suprit Malali
- Dr Nishtha Manuja
- Dr Abhinav Ahuja

Acknowledgements

Sincerely thanks to our senior post graduate resident

Dr. Vidya Hulkoti,
Dr. Nipun Bawiskar,
Dr. Gaurav Jagtap,

Dr. Twinkle Pawar,
Dr. Yash Gupte,
Dr. Amol Andhale,

Dr. Mansi Patel,
Dr. Charan Singh Bagga,
Dr. Swapnil Lahole.

Contribution by other residents cannot be ignored.

Dr. Parav Tantia,
Dr. Hamdulay Khadija,
Dr. Nikhil Reddy,
Dr. Manikanta Nelakuditi,
Dr. Mohit Gabhane,
Dr. Utkarsh Pradeep,
Dr. Ajinkya Kadu,
Dr.Nishant Rathod,
Dr. Rishabh Singh,
Dr. PreetAgrawal,
Dr. Shikha Mundra,
Dr. Adhokshaj Bhake,
Dr. Prajakta Kakde,
Dr. Viraj Wadhera,
Dr. Gankidi Raghavender,
Dr. Anusha Jha,

Dr. Harsh Babariya,
Dr. Tejas Nehete,
Dr. Manjeet Kothari,
Dr. Suhail Shaikh,
Dr. Aman Kumar Gupta,
Dr. Parepalli Avinash,
Dr. Faizan Khan,
Dr. Priyanka Negandhi,
Dr. Chetan Borse,
Dr. Maimoona Khan,
Dr. Parth Aggarwal,
Dr. Aditya Pande,
Dr. Harsh Kansagara,
Dr. Meghna Bordoloi,
Dr. AtharvRode,
Dr. Akshay Padwal,

Dr. Rushikesh Dhondge,
Dr. Navanath Deokate,
Dr. Rajvardhan Patil,
Dr. Jayanth Kumar,
Dr. Gautam Bedi,
Dr. Roma Chavhan,
Dr. Vineet Karwa,
Dr. Rushi Mukkawar,
Dr. Jaswanth Varma Alluri,
Dr. Chandranshu Vallabhaneni,
Dr. Abhimanyu Chawla,
Dr. Abhishek Ghali,
Dr. Vamshi Krishna,
Dr. Sanchit Chhabra,
Dr. Divyansh Singh,
Dr. Nidhi Bardiya.

Preamble

The faculty at Jawaharlal Nehru Medical College worked on a novel academic project, the work encompassed creating a handbook specifically elaborating on Objectively Structured Clinical Examination (OSCE).

The OSCE exercises are contributed by specialties of the Department of Medicine.

The OSCE handbook on the subject of General Medicine has been written by the curriculum and the syllabus of the subject for the final professional MBBS year and postgraduate residents. The OSCE Handbook has been put forth to have a compiled document of the OOSCE-based exercises for the subject, these exercises form a significant aspect of assessment in the practical examination.

The handbook essentially gives the student a comprehensive prototype, through which the student can have the required understanding and know-how for that particular exercise. Each OSCE write-up consists of an exercise compartmentalized into a basic introductory write-up along with steps of assessment, basic know-how, and intelligence on the experiment and its associated peripheral knowledge for a particular skill or response station. The write-up has been put forth with easy-to-understand scientific content, the flow of answers, matter, and verbatim, diagrams, concept maps, and flowcharts, all together in each of the answers. The handbook aims to instill a sense of preparedness and steadfastness among students which, in turn, would result in better outcomes and improved creativity.

The main role players of the Notebook concept are Teachers who act as the Creative end and students who then splash the best of their creativity in the form of answers.

We hope that our students have an excellent time reading the handbook and find it beneficial for their understanding of the practical exercises.

General Medicine Kit for Examination

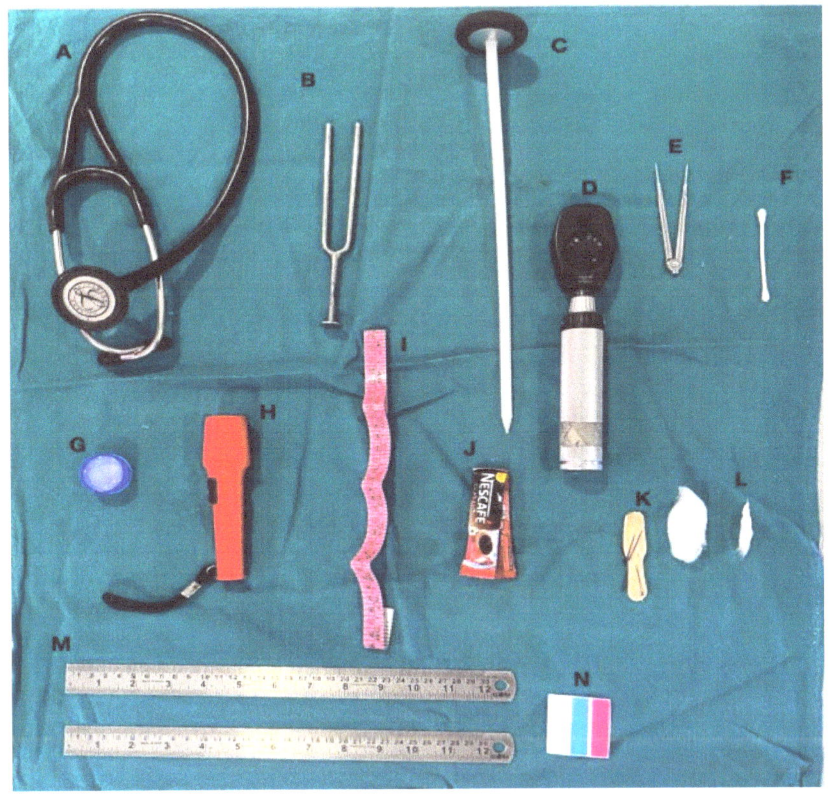

1. **Stethoscope**
2. **Tuning Fork (128 Hz)**
3. **Knee Hammer**
4. **Ophthalmoscope**
5. **Divider for Two-Point Discrimination**
6. **Cotton Bud**
7. **Mint**
8. **Torch**
9. **Measuring Tape**
10. **Coffee**
11. **Pins**
12. **Cotton**
13. **Measuring Scale**
14. **Colour strips**

Chapter 1

General Examination

General Examination

A. Pulse

Stations:

Table A.1: Checklist

Type of Station: Procedural station
Assessment of radial pulse
Domain: Cognitive, Psychomotor, Affective.
Communication Time: 1 minute   Marks: 10

No.	Steps	Marks	R No.
I	**Checklist**		
1	Stood on the Right side of the patient, made the subject comfortable in a sitting position, and explained the procedure to the patient.	1	
2	Examined the Pulse with wrist semi-flexed, forearm in the mid-prone position.	1	
3	Examined with the three fingers over the radial artery by trisection method.	1	
4	Counted the pulse for 1 minute.	1	
5	Palpated the other radial pulse simultaneously.	1	
6	Describe the pulse in rate, rhythm, volume, character, radio-radial synchronicity, radio femoral delay, and elasticity of the arterial wall.	1	
7	Examined the pulse on the other hand as well.	1	
8	Examined pulse in other arteries like carotid, femoral, popliteal, posterior tibial, and dorsalis pedis.	1	
II	**Assessment of Professional Behavior**		
1.	Addressed the patient appropriately and introduced himself/herself by name.	1	
2.	Informed patient regarding completion of the procedure and thanked the patient before leaving	1	
III	**Total Score (Tick)**	10	
	Final Score		
	Global rating: 1. Poor 2. Unsatisfactory 3. Satisfactory 4. Good 5. Excellent		
	Observer's comment (based on general observation)		
	Signature of the observer		

Introduction:

Students will be evaluated for palpation of the radial artery. The student needs to understand the clinical technique and interpretation of palpating the radial artery. Pulse is assessed in terms of rate, rhythm, volume, and character. The students will palpate the radial artery, interpret its abnormalities, and correlate it with underlying symptomatology.

Clinical application:

1. Detection of abnormalities in the examination of the radial pulse.
2. Knowledge of medical conditions associated with abnormalities in pulse.
3. Should know the physiological and pathological causes of abnormal radial pulse characteristics.

Expected from students:

1. Causes of abnormalities in rate, rhythm, volume, and character of the radial pulse.
2. The student should be aware of the required skill to assess the radial pulse
3. The student should be acquainted with the proper steps of the assessment.
4. The student needs to be aware of the expected result and its interpretation.

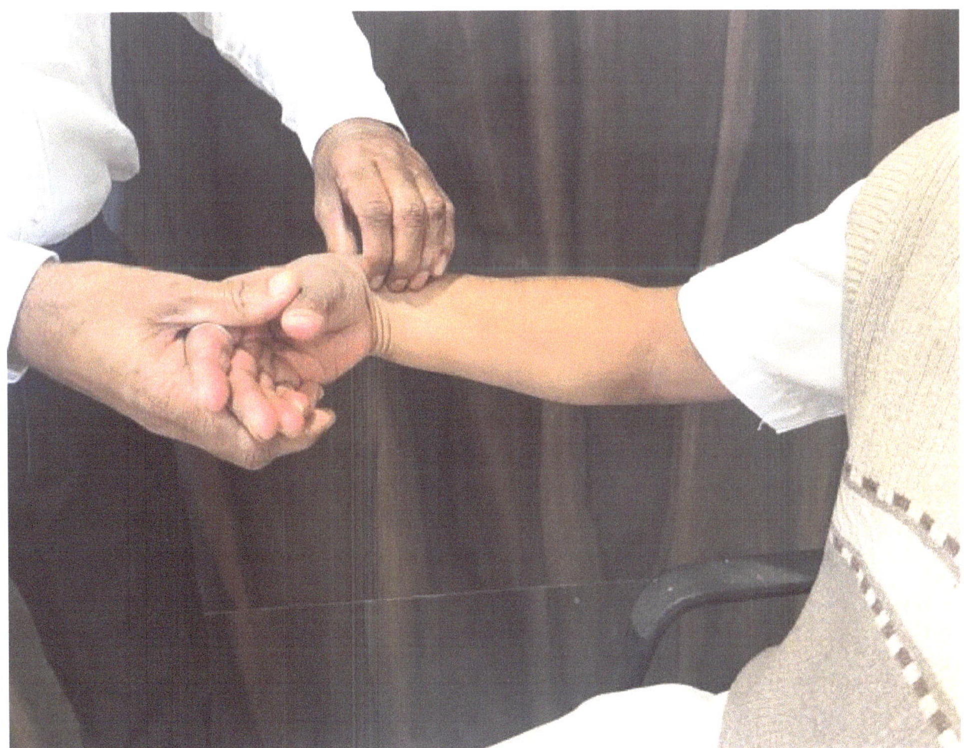

Figure A.1: Three-finger method for palpating the radial artery.

Table A.2: Different types and causes of rate, rhythm, volume, and character of pulse

Rate:

Bradycardia (<60 beats/min)	Tachycardia (>100 beats/min)
Athletes	Anxiety
Hypothyroidism	Fever
Vasovagal syncope	Pregnancy
Drugs-beta blockers	Hyperthyroidism
Heart block	Cardiac failure
Sick sinus syndrome	Tachyarrhythmias
Hypothermia	Drugs: salbutamol, terbutaline

Rhythm:

Abnormalities	Causes
Irregularly irregular	Atrial fibrillation, Frequent extrasystoles
Regular with occasional irregularity	Extra systoles
Regularly irregular	Sinus arrythmia, Pulsus bigeminus, Pulsus trigeminus, Partial AV blocks

Volume:

Hypokinetic pulse	Hyperkinetic pulse
Hypovolemia	Hyperkinetic circulation (anemia, fever, thyrotoxicosis, pregnancy)
Shock	Patent ductus arteriosus
Heart failure	Ventricular septal defect
Acute myocardial infarction	Peripheral arteriovenous fistulae
Constrictive pericarditis	Complete heart block
Mitral stenosis	Mitral regurgitation
Aortic stenosis	Aortic regurgitation

Character:

Character of pulse	Associated condition
Pulsusparvus et tardus	Aortic stenosis
Anacrotic pulse	Severe aortic stenosis
Collapsing pulse (water hammer pulse)	PDA, Aortic regurgitation, Large AV fistula, Hyperkinetic circulatory states like Anemia, Thyrotoxicosis, BeriBeri, Pregnancy
Pulsus bisferiens	Aortic stenosis + Aortic regurgitation, Severe aortic regurgitation, Hypertrophic cardiomyopathy
Dicrotic pulse	Dilated cardiomyopathy, Cardiac tamponade
Pulsus alternans	Acute left ventricular failure
Pulsus bigeminus	Coupled ectopic beats
Pulsus paradoxus	Constrictive pericarditis, Cardiac tamponade, Restrictive cardiomyopathy, Tension pneumothorax, Severe bronchial asthma

B. Blood Pressure (BP) Measurement

Table B.1: Checklist

Type of Station: measurement of blood pressure in the patient (both supine and sitting)
Domain: Cognitive, Psychomotor, Affective.
Communication Time: 1 minute

Marks-10

No.	Steps	Marks	R No.
I	**Checklist**		
1	Stood on the Right side of the patient, made the subject comfortable in a lying down position, and explained the procedure to the patient.	1	
2	Supported the patient's arm comfortably if a person was sitting.	1	
3	Positioned the bladder's center over the brachial artery when applying the cuff to the arm.	1	
4	Inflated the cuff slowly and measured Systolic Blood Pressure by palpatory method	1	
5	The cuff was inflated an additional 10 mmHg, and the brachial artery in the cubital fossa was examined with the stethoscope.	1	
6	Continued to deflate the cuff slowly until the reading of Diastolic Blood Pressure	1	
7	Mentioned the B.P. in millimeters of mercury	1	
8	Examined the blood pressure on the other hand	1	
II	**Assessment of Professional Behavior**		
1.	Addressed the patient appropriately and introduced himself/herself by name.	1	
2.	Informed patient regarding completion of the procedure and thanked the patient before leaving	1	
III	**Total Score (Tick)**	10	
	Final Score		
	Global rating: 1. Poor 2. Unsatisfactory 3. Satisfactory 4. Good 5. Excellent		
	Observer's comment (based on general observation)		
	Signature of the observer		

Introduction:

Students will be evaluated for arterial blood pressure measurement by a mercury sphygmomanometer by palpatory and auscultatory methods.

Expected from the student:

1. The student should be aware of the required instrument to measure blood pressure.
2. The student should be aware of the various other blood pressure measurement manometers.
3. The student should be well apprised of the handling of the instruments.
4. The student should be acquainted with the proper steps of the measurement.
5. The student needs to be aware of the expected result and its interpretation.

Clinical application:

1. Diagnosis of Hypertension
2. Should be knowledgeable about ambulatory blood pressure monitoring, white coat hypertension, and masked hypertension
3. Postural hypotension, which is defined as a systolic and diastolic blood pressure drop of more than 15 and 10 mmHg, respectively, when standing
4. JNC criteria for classification, interpretation, and treatment of high blood pressure.

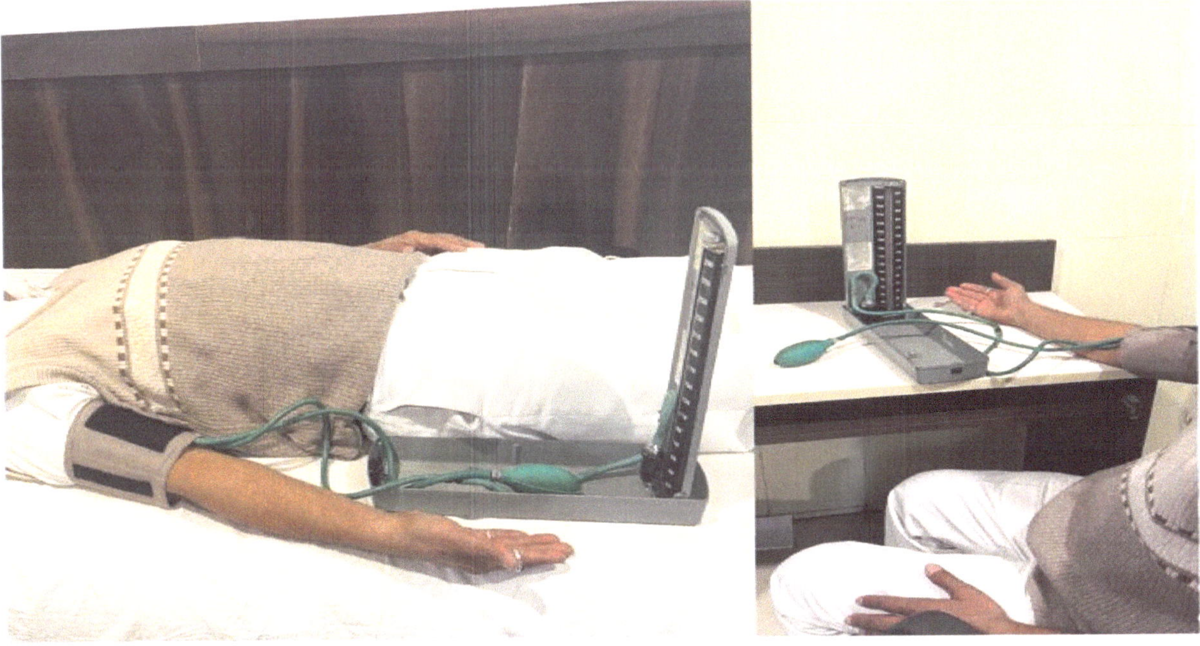

Figure B.1: Demonstrating the procedure of measuring blood pressure in supine and sitting position

Table B.2: Showing American Heart Association (AHA) Guidelines 2017

BP Category	Systolic BP	Diastolic BP
Normal BP	<120 mmHg	<80 mmHg
Elevated BP	120 – 129 mmHg	<80 mmHg
Hypertension		
Stage 1	130 – 139 mmHg	80-89 mmHg
Stage 2	140 mmHg	90 mmHg

According to the American Heart Association:

People who fall into two groups for both their systolic and diastolic blood pressure should be placed in the higher blood pressure category.

High Blood pressure is defined as based on an average of ≥2 careful readings obtained on ≥2 days of presentation to the clinician (DBP, diastolic blood pressure; and SBP, systolic blood pressure).

JNC 8 criteria:

Important changes have been made to the JNC 7 guidelines including the following:

- The target blood pressure level is now 150/90 mm Hg for patients older than 60 who don't harbor metabolic disorders such as diabetes or chronic renal disease as co-morbidities.
- New target blood pressure is kept at 140/90 mm Hg for patients between the ages of 18 and 59 without any significant coexisting conditions and for those older than 60 with diabetes, chronic kidney disease (CKD), or both.
- Diuretics of the thiazide-type, calcium channel blockers (CCBs), ACE inhibitors, and ARBs should be used as first-line and secondary therapies.

C. Pallor

Table C.1: Checklist

Type of station: General examination of pallor
Domain: Cognitive, Psychomotor, Affective.
Communication Time: 1 minute

Marks-10

Sr. no	Steps	Marks	R.no
I	**Checklist**		
1	Stood on the Right side of the patient, madethe subject comfortable in a sitting position, and explained the procedure to the patient	1	
2	Examined the patient in proper sunlight	1	
3	Looked for pallor in lower palpebral conjunctiva by asking the patient to look up and lower down the lower eyelid	1	
4	Looked in the tongue by asking to protrude out	1	
5	Examined palm and its creases	1	
6	Examined nail beds	1	
7	Looked for signs of anemia like koilonychia,platynychia, hyperpigmentation of knuckle	1	
8	Examined in both eyes as well as the hand	1	
II	**Assessment of Professional Behavior**		
1.	Addressed the patient appropriately and introduced himself/herself by name.	1	
2.	Informed patient regarding completion of the procedure and thanked the patient before leaving	1	
III	**Total Score (Tick)**	10	
	Final Score		
	Global Rating: 1. Poor; 2. Unsatisfactory; 3. Satisfactory; 4. Good; 5. Excellent		
	Observer's comment (based on general observation)		
	Signature of the observer		

Introduction:

Students should be able to identify what are the sites where we look for pallor.

Pallor is a paleness of the skin and mucosa membrane that can be caused by a reduction in the number of red blood cells in circulation or a reduction in blood flow. Pallor can be caused by anemia and vasoconstriction. Lower palpebral conjunctiva, the tongue, the palms, palmer creases, and the nail beds are common locations for the pallor.Anemia is due to hemorrhage, hemolytic, dyshemopoietic (B12 deficiency, Iron deficiency. and Folic acid deficiency).

Vasoconstriction – shock, exposure to cold,fright,syncope,atrial occlusion, cutaneous edema, Myxedema

Expected from students:

1. The student should know the definition and causes of pallor
2. The student should know the site ofthepallor examination
3. The student should know important medical causes of pallor
4. The student should know how to distinguish between similar presentations such as hypopigmentation.

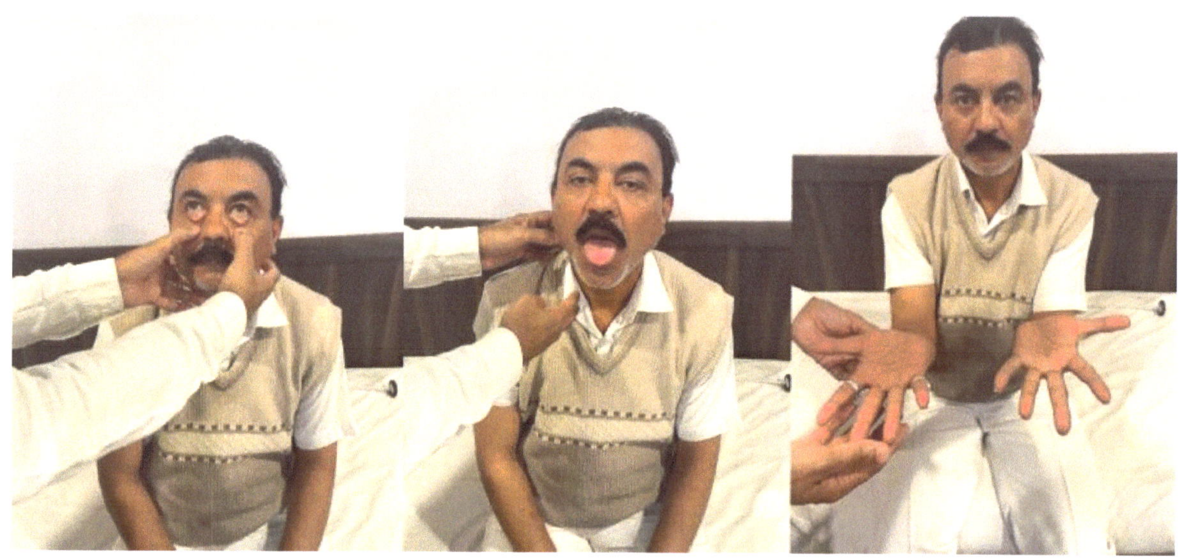

Figure C.1: Depicting the sites to look for pallor.

Clinical Application:

A strict definition of anemia is a decrease in the absolute amount of red blood cellsthat are present (a reduction in the mass of red blood cellswhich is studied by blood volume studies).

[or] Decrease in hemoglobin concentration, hematocrit (HCT), or RBC count, three of the main red blood cell (RBC) parameters acquired as part of the complete blood count (CBC), is referred to as anemia.

However, in actuality, the most common method used for this is a low hematocrit or hemoglobin concentration.

The degree of anemia, the rate at which it has developed, the patient's oxygen needs, and the signs and symptoms that anemia causes are all factors.

Slowly progressing anemia reduces the likelihood of symptoms because it gives several homeostatic mechanisms time to adapt to the blood's decreased ability to carry oxygen.

Causes of anemia:

- Iron deficiency
- B12 and folate deficiency.
- Chronic disease/inflammation
- Hemolytic anemia
- Drug-induced
- Myelodysplastic
- Aplastic anemia
- Microangiopathic hemolytic anemia

D. Icterus

Table D.1: Checklist

Type of Station: Examination of icterus in the patient
Domain: Cognitive, Psychomotor, Affective.
Communication Time: 1 minute

Marks-10

Sr. no.	Steps	Marks	R.no
I	**Checklist**		
1	Stood on the Right side of the patient and explained the procedure to the patient.	1	
2	Ensured adequate daylight.	1	
3	Examined the sclera by asking the patient to look down.	1	
4	Examined the dorsum of the tongue inthe oral cavity by asking the patients to touch the hard palate by the tip of the tongue.	2	
5	Examined skin.	1	
6	Examined nails.	1	
7	Examined in both the eyes.	1	
II	**Assessment of Professional Behavior:**		
1.	Addressed the patient appropriately and introduced himself/herself by name.	1	
2.	Informed patient regarding completion of the procedure and thanked the patient before leaving.	1	
III	**Total Score (Tick)**	**10**	
	Final Score		
	Global Rating: 1. Poor; 2. Unsatisfactory; 3. Satisfactory; 4. Good; 5. Excellent		
	Observer's comment (based on general observation)		
	Signature of the Observer		

Introduction:

Icterus is a yellowish discoloration of the skin and mucous membrane that is caused by hyperbilirubinemia and bile pigment deposition in elastin-rich tissue. Jaundice manifests clinically as icterus in people with blood bilirubin levels greater than 2-3 mg/dl.

Expected from a student:

1. Must know the classification and interpretation of icterus
2. Students should be aware of the site of examination for icterus
3. Students should be acquainted with the proper steps of the examination

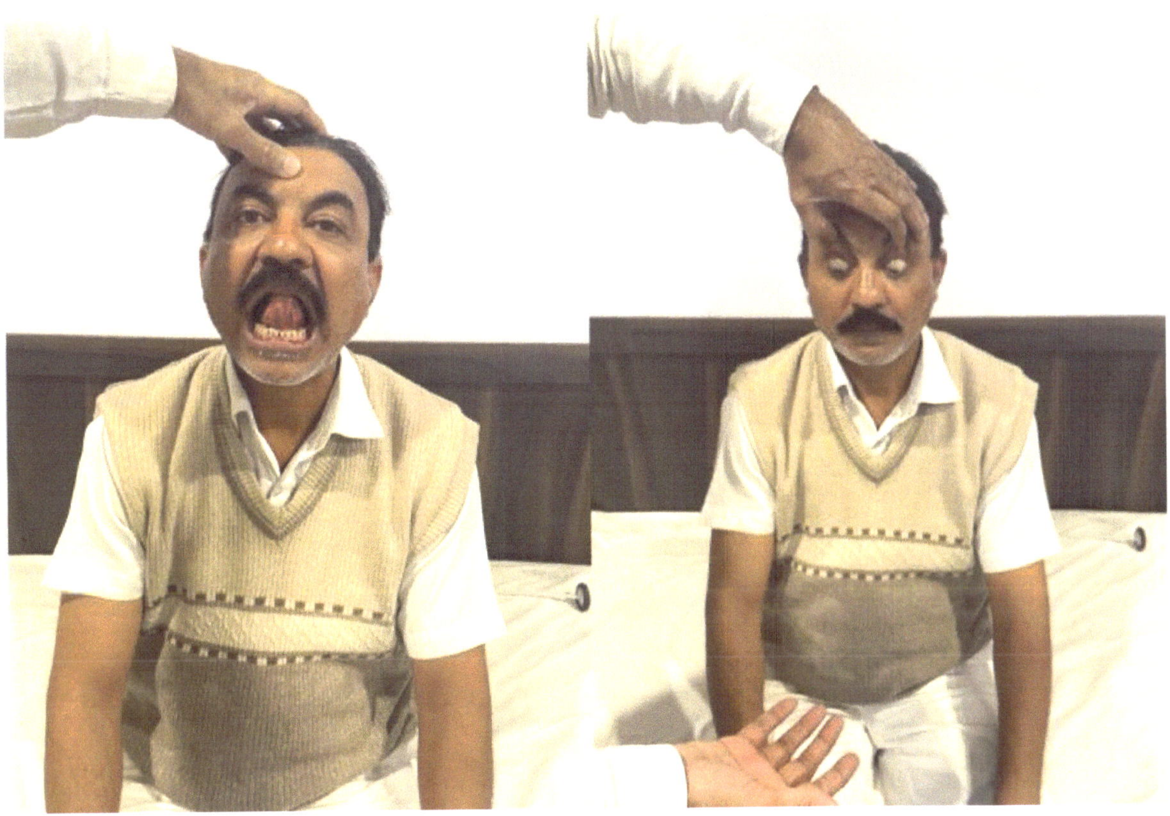

Figure D.1: Demonstrating the sites to look for icterus

Clinical application:

1. Diagnosis of icterus
2. Knowledge of various medical conditions that are diagnosed by icterus
3. Should know about hemolytic, hepatic, and obstructive jaundice

Table D.2: Showing characteristics of different types of jaundice

FEATURES	HEMOLYTIC JAUNDICE	HEPATOCELLULAR JAUNDICE	EXTRAHEPATIC CHOLESTATIC JAUNDICE
Color of urine	Normal	High colored	High colored
Color of stools	Normal	Normal to dark	Pale colored
Pruritus	-	-/+	++
Jaundice	Lemon yellow	Deep Yellow	Orange yellow/greenish yellow
Antecedent History	History of anemia requiring blood transfusions	Injection/Blood transfusion/tattoos	Biliary Surgery or gall stones
Family History	Anemia	Jaundice	Gall stones
Urine urobilinogen	Present	Present	-
Haemogram	Evidence of hemolysis	Normal	Normal
Serum Bilirubin	Unconjugated raised	Mixed	Conjugated raised
Serum Transaminases	Normal	Raised	Normal
Alkaline Phosphate	Normal	Normal/Raised	Raised

E. Clubbing

Table E.1: Checklist

Type of Station: Examination of Clubbing
Domain: Cognitive, Psychomotor, Affective.
Communication Time: 1 minute

Marks-10

Sr. no	Steps	Marks	R.no
I	**Checklist**		
1	Stand on the right side of the subject and make the subject comfortable in a sitting position and explain the procedure.	1	
2	Felt for softening at nail beds	1	
3	Saw tangentially for the obliteration of the angle between the nail & nail bed	1	
4	Looked for Lovibond's sign	1	
5	Looked for Schamroth's sign	1	
6	Examined for arthropathy	1	
7	Looked on the other hand as well	1	
8	Examined the feet for clubbing	1	
II	**Assessment of Professional Behavior**		
1	Addressed the patient appropriately and introduced himself/herself by name	1	
2	Informed patient regarding completion of the procedure and thanked the patient before leaving	1	
III	**Total Score (Tick)**	10	
	Final Score		
	Global Rating: 1. Poor; 2. Unsatisfactory; 3. Satisfactory; 4. Good; 5. Excellent		
	Observer's comment (based on general observation)		
	Signature of the Observer		

Introduction:

A digit's terminal phalanx swells uniformly and bulbously, and the normal Lovibond's angle(150 – 160 degrees) between the nail and nail bed is obliterated.

Interstitial edema and the enlargement of the arterioles and capillaries cause the terminal phalanx to expand.

Hypoxia is assumed to be the catalyst for clubbing, while the exact process is uncertain. Deep arterio-venous fistulas brought on by hypoxia increase blood flow to the fingers and toes, resulting in their enlargement.

Vascular endothelial growth factor is another important element in the physical alterations brought on by clubbing.

Expected from students:

1.   The student should know about the basic mechanism of clubbing and, the different conditions leading to clubbing.
2.   Students should be aware of the various stages/grades of clubbing.

Diagnosis of clubbing-

The proximal nail fold and nail plate form a sharp angle known as the Lovibond's angle when the distal digit is held with the finger at eye level by the examiner. It is usually less than or equal to 160 degrees. More than 160 degrees of the normal angle is lost when clubbing. 180 degrees or more is considered clubbing.

Fluctuation test: The index finger of the patient is kept on both thumbs of the examiner, stabilized by holding at distal interphalangeal joints by the middle finger (of the examiner), and then fluctuation is tested by both index fingers. [Figure 5.1]

When the tips of the fingers on both hands are facing towards one another, the steep angle that is present between the beds of the nailandthecuticle creates a hole that is diamond in shape, which is Schamroth's sign (commonly seen in index fingers). It's called Schamroth's sign when this gap closes. [Figure 5.2]

Hypertrophic osteoarthropathy(HOA): figure 5.3. – Clubbing of the digits, Periostitis of the long bones, and arthritis. [also known as pachydermoperiostosis.]

Clinical application:

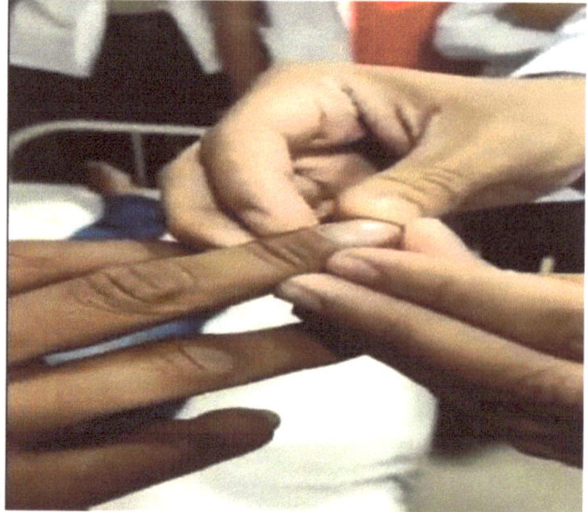

Figure E.1: Demonstrating fluctuation test

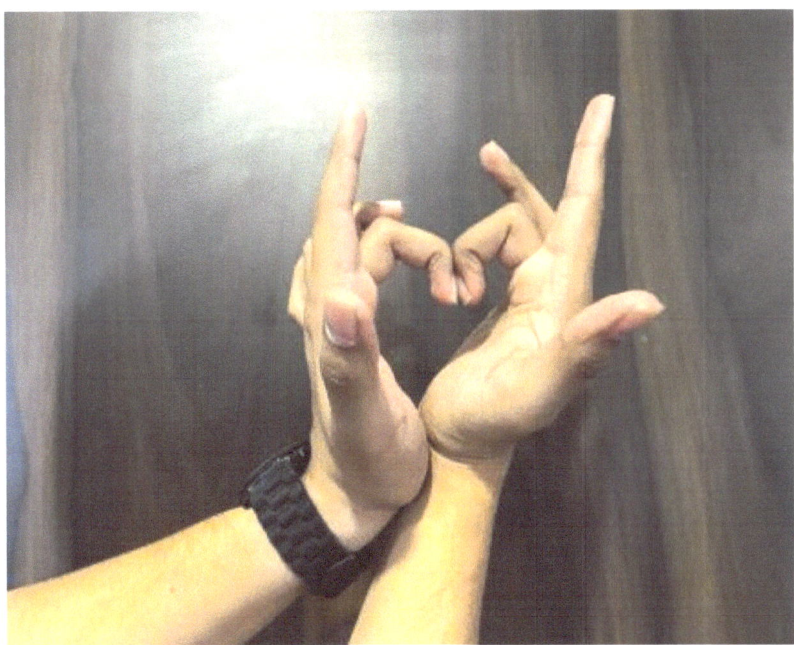

Figure E.2: Demonstrating the procedure for Schamroth's sign

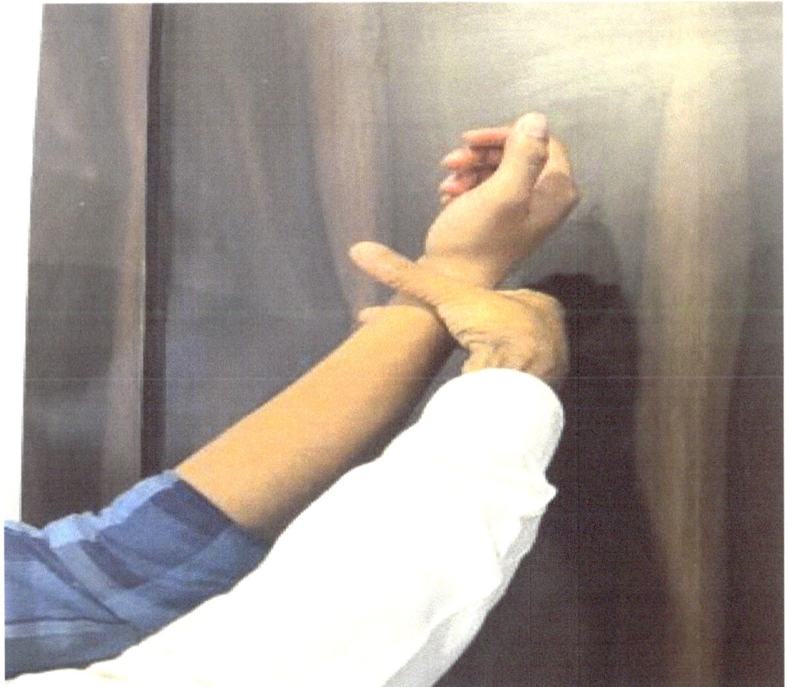

Figure E.3: Demonstrating the procedure to look for hypertrophic osteoarthropathy

Stages of clubbing:

Stage I: Normal appearance and angle but increased fluctuation of the nail bed.

Stage II: Loss of angle between nail and nail bed.

Stage III: Increased curvature of angle.

Stage IV: Expansion of terminal phalanx drum stick appearance.

Various causes of clubbing:

Pulmonary:

- Bronchogenic carcinoma, mesothelioma
- Lung abscess
- Bronchiectasis
- Tuberculosis with secondary infection
- Empyema

Cardiac:

- Infective endocarditis
- Cyanotic congenital heart disease, Eisenmenger's physiology
- Atrial myxoma

Alimentary:

- Ulcerative Colitis
- Crohn'sDisease
- Hepato – Pulmonary Syndrome

Endocrine:

- Myxoedema
- Acromegaly

Table F.1: Checklist

Type of Station: Eliciting the examination of Lymphadenopathy.

Domain: Cognitive, Psychomotor, Affective.

Communication Time: 1 minute

Marks-10

Sr.no	Steps	Marks	R.no
I	**Checklist**		
1	Stands in front of the subject and makes the subject comfortable in a sitting position and explains the procedure.	1	
2	Stands in front of the patient for examination of the posterior group of lymph nodes (Occiput, behind the ear, retro auricular, Posterior triangle, Jugulodigastric).	1	
3	Stands behind the patient to look for an anterior group of lymph nodes (Sub Mental, Sub Mandibular, Anterior triangle, Anterior to Jugulodigastric muscle).	1	
4	Palpates the scalene group of lymph nodes by the thumb and index finger behind the sternal head of the sternocleidomastoid muscle.	1	
5	Palpates the axillary group of lymph nodes by slight abduction of the arm (Anterior group in the anterior axillary fold, Posterior group in the posterior axillary fold, lateral group, central group by insinuating the finger at the apex).	2	
6	Looked for epitrochlear lymph node, by flexing elbow joint at 90 degrees.	1	
7	Repeat the procedure in the other arm.	1	
II	**Assessment of Professional Behavior**		
1	Addressed the patient appropriately and introducedhimself/herself by name.	1	
2	Informed patient regarding completion of the procedure and thanked the patient before leaving.	1	
III	**Total Score (Tick)**	10	
	Final score		
	Global Rating: 1. Poor; 2. Unsatisfactory; 3. Satisfactory; 4. Good; 5. Excellent		
	Observer's comment (based on general observation)		
	Signature of the Observer		

Introduction:

Students will be evaluated for demonstration of Lymphadenopathy. The student needs to understand the clinical technique and interpretation of Lymphadenopathy. The size and consistency are of utmost importance when looking out for lymphadenopathy.

Expected from a student:

- The student should be acquainted with the proper steps of the examination of lymphadenopathy.
- The student needs to be aware of the expected result and its interpretation.

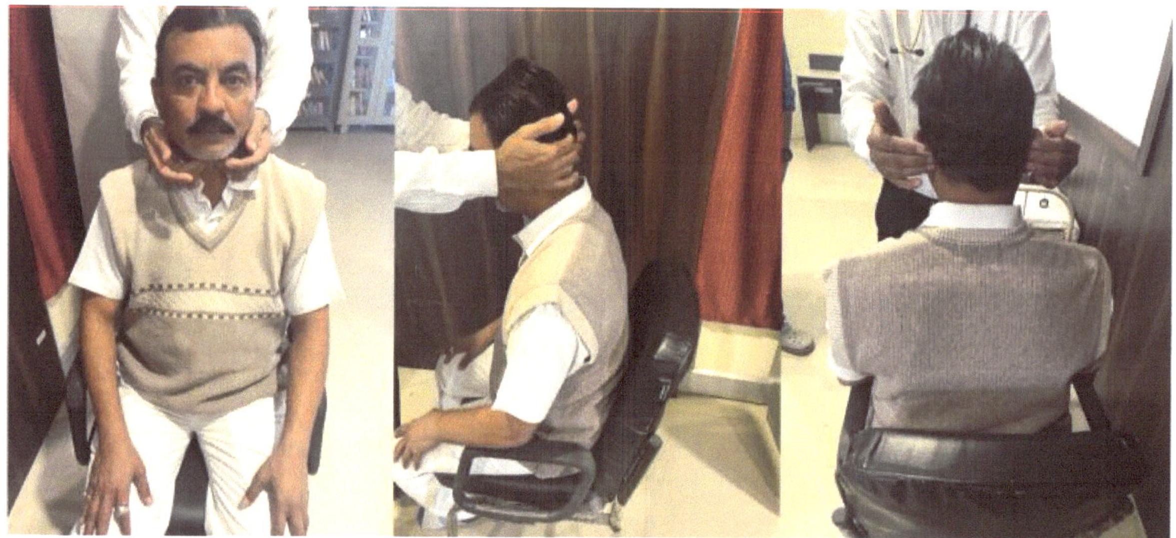

Figure F.1: Demonstrating the method to look for lymphadenopathy

Clinical application:

- Know the causes of Lymphadenopathy.
- Assessment and interpretation of Lymphadenopathy.

Lymphadenopathy:

- When two or more lymph node groups are affected, it is called generalized lymphadenopathy.
- The term used to describe the presence of lymph nodes larger than 1 cm in size in two or more regions for longer than three months is persistent generalized lymphadenopathy.
- Lymph nodes are described according to size, site, number, consistency, mobility, and tenderness.
- Important terms in the description of Lymphadenopathy--
- Normal – Soft
- Malignant – Hard
- Lymphoma – Rubber in consistency
- Tuberculosis – Matted (due to periadenitis)

The common causes of generalized lymphadenopathy are:

- Tuberculosis
- HIV
- Infectious mononucleosis
- Malignancies like Lymphomas, Acute and Chronic Leukemias
- Granulomatosis, Sarcoidosis
- Kikuchi – Fujimoto disease
- Kimura disease
- Rheumatological conditions like SLE, JRA, and Sjogrens syndrome

There are two types of cervical lymph nodes: superficial and deep. Submental, submandibular, preauricular, postauricular, occipital, paratracheal, paratracheal, and posterior triangles are among the superficial lymph node groupings.

Supraclavicular, scalene, Jugulo – digastric, and Jugulo – Omohyoid lymph nodes are deep cervical lymph nodes.

The axillary group of lymph nodes includes Lateral, Anterior, Posterior, Central, and Apical groups.

Examination of Cervical Lymph nodes:

- Standing behind the patient and flexing the neck to look for the submental group, submandibular group, pre-auricular group, jugulo-digastric and jugulo-omohyoid, and finally supraclavicular groups during the examination of the anterior group of lymph nodes.
- Standing in front of the patient, the examiner starts by looking for the post-auricular lymph nodes, then the occipital, and finally the posterior group of lymph nodes.

G. Jugular Venous Pressure

Table G.1: Checklist

Type of Station: Measurement of jugular venous pressure (JVP) in the patient.
Domain: Cognitive, Psychomotor, Affective.
Communication Time: 1 minute

Marks-10

Sr. no	Steps	Marks	R.no
I	**Checklist**		
1	Stood on the Right side of the patient and explained the procedure to the patient	1	
2	Exposed neck and chest of the subject (up to sternal angle).	1	
3	Makes the subject comfortable in a 45-degree position by providing a backrest.	1	
4	Asked the patients to look towards the left, and look for internal jugular vein pulsation in the area made by the two heads of the sternomastoid muscle (clavicular and sternal).	1	
5	Marked the two-point (angle of Louis/sternal angle and upper level of IJV pulsation.	1	
6	Measure the JVP properly by taking the help of two scales. The upper level of venous pulsation by the horizontal scale and vertical scale at the sternal angle.	1	
7	Measure the JVP by adding 5cm.	1	
8	Perform hepatojugular reflux if JVP is not visualized.	1	
II	**Assessment of Professional Behavior**		
1.	Addressed the patient appropriately and introduced himself/herself by name.	1	
2.	Informed patient regarding completion of the procedure and Thanked the patient before leaving	1	
III	**Total Marks (Tick)**	10	
	Final score		
	Global Rating: 1. Poor; 2. Unsatisfactory; 3. Satisfactory; 4. Good; 5. Excellent		
	Observer's comment (based on general observation)		
	Signature of the Observer		

Introduction:

- Students will be evaluated for demonstration of Jugular Venous Pressure.
- The student needs to understand the clinical technique, and interpretation of Jugular Venous Pressure and the various waveforms associated with it.
- An indirect way to quantify central venous pressure is by the demonstration of jugular venous pressure.
- Changes in right atrial pressure are reflected in the internal jugular vein (IJV), which is more frequently employed because it links to the right atrium without any intervening valves and produces a continuous column of blood (e.g. raised right atrial pressure results in distension of the IJV).
- When doing a clinical assessment, the external jugular vein (EJV) is frequently utilized as a stand-in for measuring central venous pressure (as IJV is difficult to visualize, though EJV is a less reliable indicator as it passes through muscle fascia and has multiple valves).
- JVP is found in the fossa formed by the sternal and clavicular heads of the sternomastoid muscle after the person is placed in a 450 semi-recumbent position with the neck slightly curved to the left.
- The JVP is difficult to palpate and features a double waveform pulse (i.e., two pulses) (helps to distinguish between carotid pulsations and JVP).

Differentiate from carotid arterial pulsation:

- After the JVP has been located, the vertical distance between Louis' angle and the JVP's most cranial point is measured using a different ruler that is inserted at a right angle to Louis' angle (+5 is added to the measured value since it is the distance between the sternal angle and right atrium).
- The hepatojugular/abdominojugular reflex: It is induced by applying sustained, firm pressure for at least 10 seconds over the right upper quadrant of the abdomen. A rise of more than 3 cm in JVP that continues for at least 15 seconds after the hand is released is considered a favorable reaction. Patients must be instructed not not hold their breath or use a Valsalva-like manoeuvre while the treatment is being done. In individuals with heart failure, abdominojugular reflux helps predict a pulmonary artery wedge pressure greater than 15 mmHg.

Clinical application:

1. Physiology behind different waveforms of JVP and the abnormalities of it.
2. Normal value of JVP and the causes of elevated JVP.
3. Significance of Hepatojugular reflux and Kussmaul's sign.

NOTES:

The JVP has a unique waveform with 5 components:

a wave

- The right atrium's constriction is what produces a wave.
- Clinical use: high "a" waves (seen in T.S., P.A.H., right atrial thrombus/mass), cannon "a" waves (observed with premature atrial/junctional beats, total AV block, and ventricular tachycardia). In atrial fibrillation, there is no "a."

c wave

- The right ventricle's contraction and the tricuspid valve's expansion into the right atrium are what trigger the c wave.

x descent

- Right atrial relaxation leads to the x decline.

v wave

- The right atrium relaxation while the tricuspid valve is still closed due to atrial filling, which results in the v wave.
- Clinical application: T.R. reveals a strong "v" wave.

y descent

- When the tricuspid valve opens, blood from the right atrium fills the right ventricle, which lowers the JVP, and the y descent takes place.
- Rapid 'y' descent in constrictive pericarditis is a clinical application.

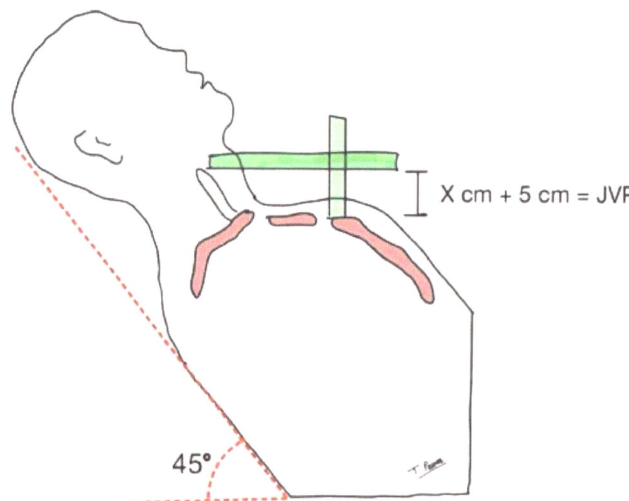

Figure G.1: Showing method to observe and measure the jugular venous pressure

JVP decreases in hypovolemia and increases in conditions such as constrictive pericarditis, pericardial compression/tamponade, pulmonary hypertension, right or left heart failure, superior vena cava obstruction, and tricuspid stenosis.

Kussmaul's sign: Neck veins rise with inspiration rather than fall, as seen with normal subjects, seen in pericardial tamponade or right heart failure.

H. Pedal Edema

Table H.1: Checklist

Type of Station: Examination of edema

Domain: Cognitive, Psychomotor, Affective.

Communication Time: 1 minute

Marks-10

Sr. no	Steps	Marks	R.no
I	**Checklist**		
1	Stood on the Right side of the patient, made subject comfortable in lying down position, and explained the procedure to the patient	1	
2	Expose both lower limbs up to the knee	1	
3	Applied pressure by thumb for 30 seconds on medial malleolus, shin of the tibia	2	
4	Looked for pitting	1	
5	Examined in both lower limbs	1	
6	Looked in other sites like sacrum in lying down (in moribund patients)	2	
II	**Assessment of Professional Behaviour**		
1	Addressed the patient appropriately and introduced himself/herself by name	1	
2	Informed patient regarding completion of the procedure and thanked the patient before leaving	1	
III	**Total Marks (Tick)**	10	
	Final Score		
	Global Rating: 1. Poor; 2. Unsatisfactory; 3. Satisfactory; 4. Good; 5. Excellent		
	Observer's comment (based on general observation)		
	Signature of the Observer		

Introduction:

The student should be able to locate the area and then palpate the pedal edema using a variety of techniques. The accumulation of extra fluid in the body's interstitium from the intravascular components is known as pedal edema. Edema can be classified as generalized (Anasarca), localized, quick, or slow.

Clinical Application:

1. Diagnosing edema
2. Understanding the causes of edema
3. Correlating gradations of edema with underlying condition
4. Knowledge of various medical conditions that cause edema

Physical examination:

Bilateral edema can be caused by a local cause or a systemic condition such as congestive heart failure, chronic kidney disease, or nephrotic syndrome.

Unilateral leg edema is typically caused by local causes such as Deep Vein Thrombosis (DVT), venous insufficiency, or lymphedema.

Lipidemia causes the dorsum of the foot to be spared, yet lymphedema and pain prominently involve it.

DVT and lipidemia are often tender, and lymphedema is usually non-tender.

DVT, venous insufficiency, early lymphedema, myxedema and the advanced fibrotic forms of lymphedema often do not pit.

Sign of Kaposi stimmer (inability to pinch a fold of skin on the dorsum of the foot at the base of the second toe is a sign of lymphedema).

The students in this particular procedural station will demonstrate the edema through various methodologies, as well as various gradations of edema.

Expected from students:

1. The student should know the definition and causes of edema
2. The student should know how to examine pedal edema
3. The student should know how to differentiate between pitting and non-pitting edema.
4. The student should know the approach to a case of edema

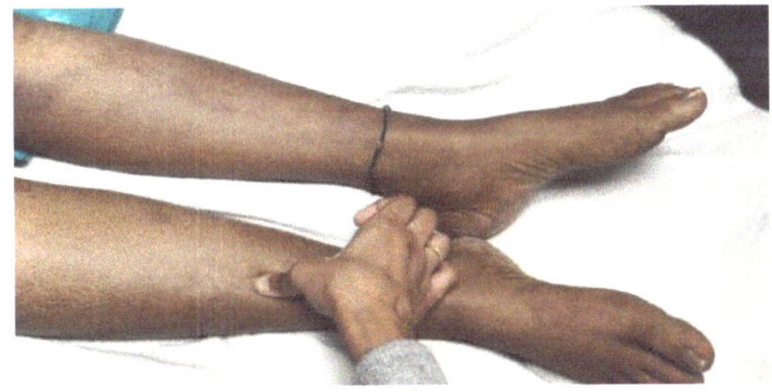

Figure H.1:-Showing pitting pedal edema.

Chapter 2

Central Nervous System

Systemic Examination

A. Cranial Nerves (Olfactory Nerve)

a. First Cranial Nerve (Olfactory Nerve)

Table A.a.1: Checklist

Type of Station: Eliciting the examination of Olfaction
Domain: Cognitive, Psychomotor, Affective.
Communication Time: 1 minute

Marks-10

Sr. no	Steps	Marks	R.no
I	**Checklist**		
1	Stood in front of the patient,madethesubject comfortable in a sitting position, and explained the procedure to the patient	1	
2	The examiner should be equipped with a familiar compound like soap, to be used for the examination	2	
3	Ask the patient to close the eyes	1	
4	Ask the patient to close one nostril and take the testing compound to the other nostril and ask to identify the compound	2	
5	Looked for both the nostrils which should not be full of secretions	1	
6	Repeats the procedure in the other nostril	1	
II	**Assessment of Professional Behavior**		
1	Addressed the patient appropriately and introduced himself/herself by name	1	
2	Informed patient regarding completion of the procedure and thanked the patient before leaving	1	
III	**Total Marks (Tick)**	10	
	Final Score		
	Global Rating: 1. Poor; 2. Unsatisfactory; 3. Satisfactory; 4. Good; 5. Excellent		
	Observer's comment (based on general observation)		
	Signature of the Observer		

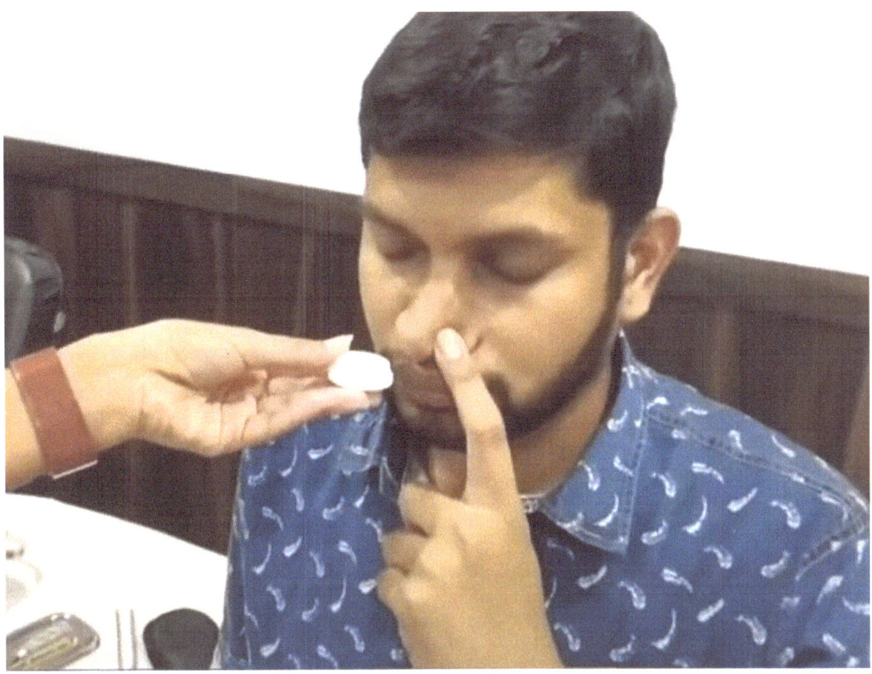

Figure A.a.1: Demonstrating the method to test the olfactory nerve.

Introduction:

Students will be evaluated for demonstration of Olfaction testing with the help of substances like Peppermint and coffee beans. The student needs to understand the clinical technique and interpretation of the olfaction. The olfaction is mediated by the First Cranial Nerve or the Olfactory Nerve. The student should understand the olfactory pathway and should know the important causes of Anosmia.

Expected from a student:

- The student should be acquainted with the proper steps of eliciting the examination of olfaction.
- The student needs to be aware of the expected result and its interpretation.

Clinical application:

- Eliciting the olfactory examination
- Knowledge of causes of anosmia
- The olfactory pathway
- Syndromes associated with Anosmia

Notes:

Olfactory Nerve:

The Olfactory Nerve is the first Cranial nerve. It is a sensory nerve with a single function – Olfaction. It is the only nerve that does not go through the thalamus and also does not go through the brainstem.

Procedure: The sense of smell is tested using non-irritating stimuli. It is tested using substances like Coffee, Cinnamon, and Peppermint. Each nostril is tested separately while occluding the other.

The patient is asked to close their eyes. The test substance is brought near the open nostril and the patient is asked whether he can identify the smell and name the substance that is being tested. Repeat the same with another substance on the other nostril. The abnormal side is to be tested first.

Table A.a.2: Olfaction Abnormalities

Anosmia	No sense of smell
Hyposmia	A decrease in the sense of smell
Hypersomnia	An overly acute sense of smell
Dysosmia	Impairment in the sense of smell
Parosmia	Distortion of smell/Perversion of smell
Phantosmia	Perception of odor that is not real
Cacosmia	Inappropriately disagreeable odors
Olfactory Agnosia	Inability to identify the detected odors

Local causes of Anosmia

- Acute Rhinitis
- Heavy Smoking
- Atrophy of Bulb

Systemic causes of Anosmia

- Vitamin B12 deficiency
- Chronic Kidney Disease
- Refsum's disease
- Parkinsonism
- Meningitis
- Intracranial tumors
- Diabetes Mellitus, Hypothyroidism

Syndromes associated with Anosmia

Foster Kennedy Syndrome: Anosmia, Optic Atrophy of one eye, and Papilledema in the other eye (due to an Intracranial tumor)

Pseudo Foster Kennedy Syndrome: Anosmia, Optic Atrophy of one eye, and Papilledema in the other eye (In the absence of an Intracranial tumor)

Kallaman syndrome: Anosmia/hyposmia and isolated hypogonadotropichypogonadism. Due to gonadotropin-releasing hormone deficiency.

b. Second Cranial nerve (optic nerve)

Table A.b.1: Checklist

Type of Station: Eliciting the examination of Vision
Domain: Cognitive, Psychomotor, Affective.
Communication Time: 1 minute   Marks-10

Sr. no	Steps	Marks	R.no
I	**Checklist**		
1	Stood in front of the subject and madethesubject comfortable in a sitting position and explained the procedure.	1	
2	The examiner should be equipped with the tools to be used for examination like a pin with a redhead and an Ishihara chart	1	
3	The patient is tested by asking him to count the fingers from a distance of one foot.	1	
4	Ask the patient to read the written material with one eye closed and repeat the same in the other eye	1	
5	The patient is tested for color vision	1	
6	The patient is tested for visual perimetry by Confrontation test by sitting in front of the patient at a distance of one foot. The patient is asked to close one eye and the examiner closes the opposite eye by sitting in front of the patient. The fingers are brought from all the quadrants temporally to nasally. It is repeated in the other eye.	1	
7	The patient is tested for Pupillary reflex by looking for the constriction of the pupil in the same eye and is also tested for the constriction of the pupil in the opposite eye.	2	
II	**Assessment of Professional Behavior**		
1	Addressed the patient appropriately and introduced himself/herself by name	1	
2	Informed patient regarding completion of the procedure and thanked the patient before leaving	1	
III	**Total Marks (Tick)**	10	
	Final Score		
	Global Rating: 1. Poor; 2. Unsatisfactory; 3. Satisfactory; 4. Good; 5. Excellent		
	Observer's comment (based on general observation)		
	Signature of the Observer		

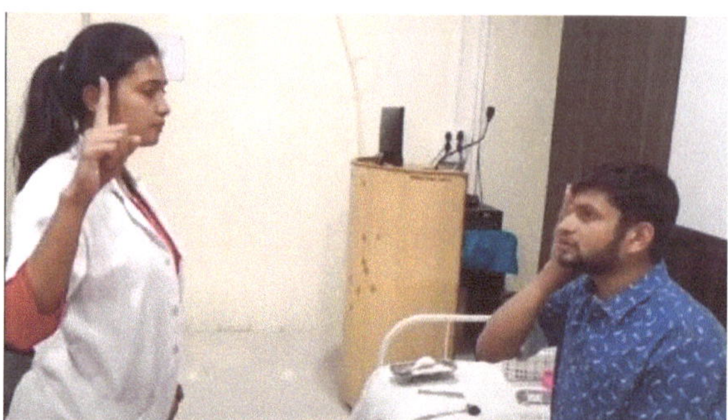

Figure A.b.1: Demonstrating the method of finger counting.

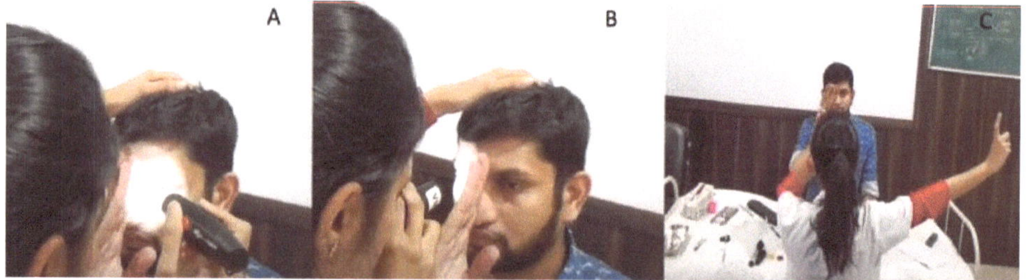

Figure A.b.2: A and B – Looking at consensual light reflex;
C – Demonstrating the method of confrontation test.

Introduction:

Students will be evaluated for demonstration of Visual acuity testing, Pupillary reflex testing, color vision testing, and confrontation test. The vision is mediated by the Second Cranial Nerve or the Optic Nerve. The student should understand the visual pathway and should know the important causes of loss of vision.

Expected from a student:

- The student should be acquainted with the proper steps of eliciting the examination of near vision, color vision, visual acuity, and light reflex.
- The student needs to be aware of the expected result and its interpretation.

Clinical application:

- Eliciting the vision examination
- Knowledge of causes of loss of vision
- The visual pathway
- Syndromes associated with vision

The Optic Nerve is the second cranial nerve responsible for Near Vision, Far Vision, and Colour vision.

It also mediates the Pupillary reflex. The light rays reach the retina on the opposite sides. Nasal light rays enter the temporal half of the retina and the temporal light rays enter the nasal half of the retina. From the retina, it is conducted through the optic nerve then, it crosses to the other half forming the optic chiasma from which the optic tract arises. From the optic tract and the lateral geniculate body arises the geniculo-calcarine tract which fans out and ends at the Primary Visual area (the striate cortex).

Procedure: The optic nerve is tested by the following tests.

- Snellen's chart is used for testing the far vision of visual acuity. In case of unavailability of Snellens chart, finger counting is done from a distance of 6 meters.
- For near vision, a Jaeger chart is used and is examined from a distance of 30 cm.
- Colour vision is tested by using Ishihara's chart.
- Fundus examination is done by direct ophthalmoscope.

The visual field testing is done by visual perimetry which is done by the Confrontation method. In the confrontation method, the examiner sits in front of the patient at a distance of 1 meter or a distance of one full hand. To examine the right eye of the patient, the patient is asked to close the left eye with his left hand and the examiner closes his right eye with his right hand. The examiner brings the flickering left finger from the temporal extremities to the nasal extremities from all the quadrants. To test the other eye, the procedure is repeated closing the right eye of the patient with the right hand and the examiner closes the left eye with his left hand, and the procedure is repeated.

The normal extent of the visual field in binocular vision is 200 degrees horizontally and 140 degrees vertically. When examined individually, the lateral extent of vision is 100 degrees, medially 60 degrees, vertically upwards is 60 degrees, and vertically downwards is 75 degrees.

The optic nerve is also tested by the Pupillary reflex which is mediated by both the optic and oculomotor nerve.

The direct light reflex is tested by flashing the light from the lateral side of theeyeonto the pupil and is looked out for constriction of the pupil in the same eye.

Indirect light reflex is tested by flashing the light from the lateral side of one eye and the constriction of the pupil is looked for in the second eye.

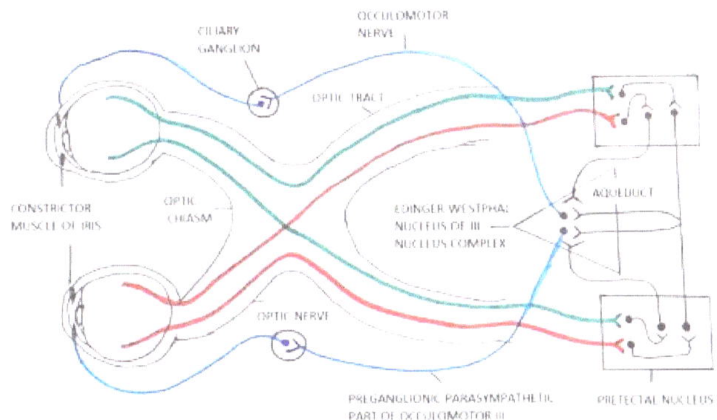

Figure A.b.3: Showing Pupillary reflex pathway

Common Causes of loss of visual acuity:

1. Refractive errors
2. Cataracts
3. Vitreous opacities

c. Third Cranial Nerve (Oculomotor Nerve)

Table A.c.1: Checklist

Type of Station: Examination of the oculomotor nerve
Domain: Cognitive, Psychomotor, Affective
Communication Time: 1 minute

Marks-10

Sr. No.	Steps	Marks	R.no
I	**Checklist**		
1	Stood on the Right Side of the patient and explained the procedure to the patient.	1	
2	Ensured adequate daylight.	1	
3	Examined eyelids.	1	
4	Examined eyes for squint.	1	
5	Examined all ranges of extraocular movements.	2	
6	Examined pupils and nystagmus.	1	
7	Commented on the presence/absence of CN III palsy and thanked the patient.	1	
II	**Assessment of Professional Behavior**		
1	Addressed the patient appropriately and Introduced himself/herself by name	1	
2	Informed patient regarding completion of the procedure and thanked the patient before leaving	1	
III	**Total Marks (Tick)**	10	
	Final Score		
	Global Rating: 1. Poor; 2. Unsatisfactory; 3. Satisfactory; 4. Good; 5. Excellent		
	Observer's comment (based on general observation)		
	Signature of the Observer		

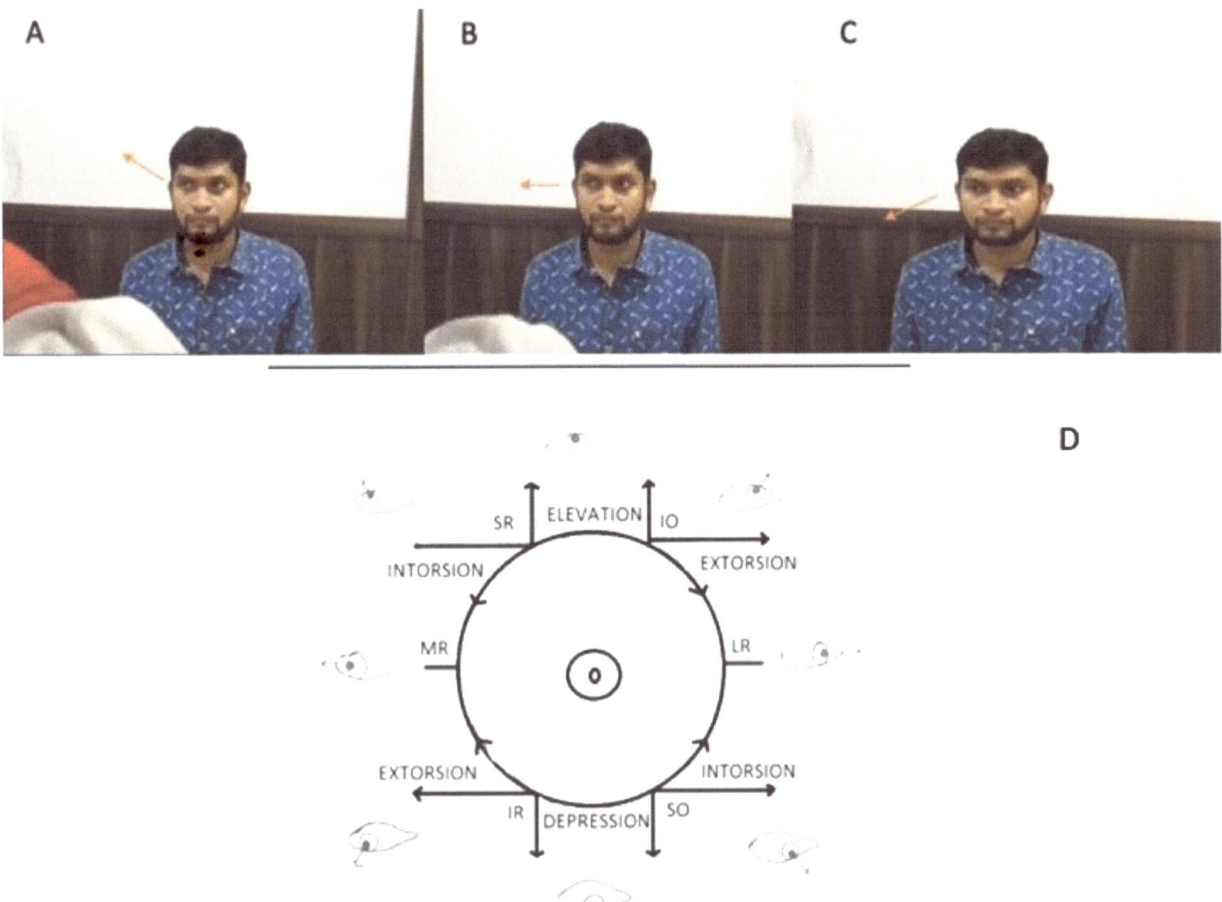

Figure A.c.1-A: Looking for the superior rectus of the right eye and inferior oblique of the left eye; **B:** Looking for the functioning of lateral rectus muscle in the right eye and medial rectus in the left eye; **C:** Looking for the right inferior rectus and left superior oblique muscle functioning; **D:** Graphic presentation of all the muscle

Introduction:

The oculomotor nerve is the third cranial nerve arising from the midbrain and supplies the extra ocular muscles of the eye except for the lateral rectus and superior oblique which are supplied by the 6th and 4th cranial nerve respectively. It also supplies the sphincter pupillae and ciliary muscles. The examination will be done in terms of the following headings:

Eyelids
Eyeballs at rest
Extraocular muscle movements
Pupils
Nystagmus

Expected From Students:

1. Guidelines for classification and interpretation of oculomotor nerve functions.
2. Students should be aware of the site of examination for the oculomotor nerve.
3. Students should be acquainted with the proper steps of the examination

Clinical application:

1. Diagnosis of CN III palsy.
2. Knowledge of various conditions leading to CN III palsy.
3. Should know the nerve supply of extraocular muscles, squint, pupillary reflex pathway, and internal/external ophthalmoplegia.

Brief summary:

1. Ptosis: Ptosis can be due to congenital or acquired. Acquired ptosis can be neurogenic, neuromuscular, myogenic, or mechanical. Oculomotor nerve lesion caused neurogenic ptosis by paralyzing LPS muscle. There is wrinkling of the forehead due to voluntary contraction of the frontalis muscle. Oculomotor nerve palsy generally causes unilateral ptosis.
2. Eyeballs at rest: Oculomotor nerve lesions generally do not cause exophthalmos or enophthalmos. However, Horner's syndrome can be ruled out.
3. Extraocular muscles: Except lateral rectus and superior oblique, all remaining muscles are supplied by CN III. CN III palsy to the 'down and out' position of the eyeball.
4. Light reflex:

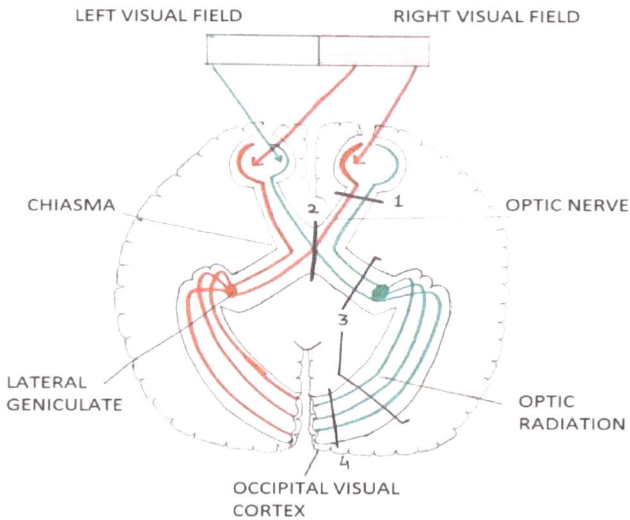

Figure A.c.2: Shows that the efferent limb of the light reflex is through the CN III. Thus, CN III palsy leads to large pupils (mydriasis).

5. Nystagmus: Nystagmus is involuntary, conjugate, repetitive, and rhythmic movements of the eyeball. CN III lesion generally does not present with nystagmus unless there is an underlying central pathology.

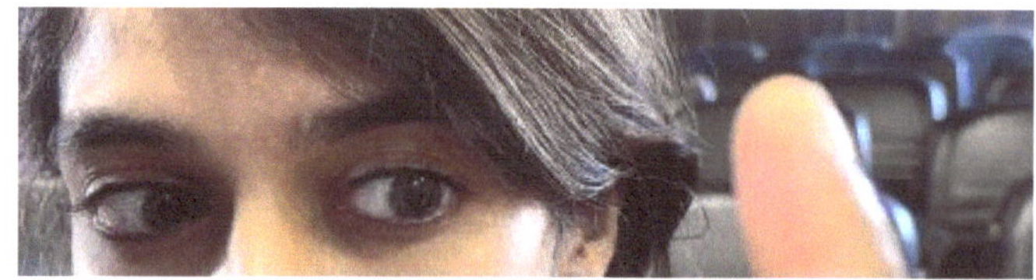

Figure A.c.3: Demonstrating the method to examine for nystagmus

d. Fourth and Sixth Cranial Nerves (Trochlear and Abducens Nerve)

Table A.d.1: Checklist

Type of Station: Eliciting the examination of the Trochlear and abducens nerve
Domain: Cognitive, Psychomotor, Affective.
Communication Time: 1 minute   Marks-10

Sr. no	Steps	Marks	R. No
I	**Checklist**		
1	Stands in front of the subject and makes the subject comfortable and explains the procedure.	1	
2	Ask the patient to look medially and downwards and then laterally	1	
3	Looked for the primary function like intorsion	2	
4	Looked for secondary functions like looking down	2	
5	Looked for tertiary functions like abduction	1	
6	Examined the other eye as well	1	
II	**Assessment of professional behavior**		
1	Addressed the patient appropriately and introduced himself/herself by name.	1	
2	Informs patient regarding completion of the procedure and thanks the subject.	1	
III	**Total Marks (Tick)**	10	
	Final Score		
	Global Rating: 1. Poor; 2. Unsatisfactory; 3. Satisfactory; 4. Good; 5. Excellent		
	Observer's comment (based on general observation)		
	Signature of the Observer		

Introduction:

The 4th cranial nerve or the Trochlear nerve has pure somatic motor function.

The trochlear nucleus gives rise to this nerve.

It goes forward and downwards in the subarachnoid space before piercing the dura mater which is close to the sphenoid bone's clinoid process.

The nerve then follows the lateral wall of the cavernous sinus.

It then enters the subarachnoid space to travel in the area which is known as Dorello's canal.

At the tip of the petrous temporal bone, this abducens nerve leaves Dorello's canal and then enters the cavernous sinus which is a dural venous sinus.

It then travels through the cavernous sinus and then enters the bony orbit through the superior orbital fissure.

Within the bony orbit, the abducens nerve terminates by innervating the lateral rectus muscle.

The lateral rectus 6thnerve (LR-6) – moves the eye horizontally outwards. The medial rectus (Bird nerve) – moves the eye horizontally inwards. The superior rectus (third nerve) – elevates the eye when it is turnedoutwards. The inferior oblique (third nerve) – elevates the eye when it is turned inwards. The inferior rectus (third nerve) – depresses the eye when it is turned outwards. The superior oblique (IVth nerve SO-4) – depresses the eye when it is turned inwards.

Clinical Application:

Trochlear nerve palsy commonly presents with vertical diplopia exacerbated while looking downwards and inwards (such as when reading or while walking downwards and inwards. Patients can also develop a head tilt away from the side which is affected.

Causes of abducens nerve palsy are the following:

- Space occupying lesion
- Diabetic neuropathy
- Cavernous sinus thrombosis

Clinical features of abducens nerve palsy:

- Diplopia
- Inability to abduct the eye for which patient rotate their head to look sideways

Table A.d.2 – Common causes of third nerve involvement

Site	Common Causes	Nerves Involved
Brainstem	Stroke (ischemic/hemorrhagic) Demyelination Interracial neoplasm	Third – mid-brain VIth – Pontomedullary junction
Meningeal	Meningitis Raised intracranial pressure Aneurysms Cerebellopontine angle tumor Trauma	IIIrd,IVth, and VIth VIth,IIIrd (uncal herniation) IIIrd (posterior communicating artery aneurysm) VIth IIIrd,IVth, and VIth
Cavernous Sinus	Infection/Thrombosis Aneurysm Caroticocavernous fistula	IIIrd,IVth, and VIth
Superior orbital fissure	Granuloma,tumor	IIIrd, IVth, and VIth
Orbit	Ischemic (diabetes,vasculitis)	IIIrd, IVth and VIth

e. Fifth Cranial Nerve (Trigeminal nerve)

Table A.e.1: Checklist

Type of Station: Procedural station

Demonstrating trigeminal nerve examination in the patient

Domain: Cognitive, Psychomotor, Affective.

Communication Time: 1 minute Marks-10

Sr. no	Steps	Marks	Roll.no
A	**Checklist**		
1	Stand on the right side of the subjectandmakethesubject comfortable in a sitting position and explain the procedure.	1	
2	Apply cotton wisp on both sides of the forehead, cheek, and chin near the midline.	1	
3	Inspect the symmetry of the angle of the jaw on both sides and watch for the hollowing of the temporal fossa.	1	
4	Put hands anterior to the tragus on both sides and watch for the movement of both hands.	1	
5	Put the hand under the jaw and ask the patient to open their mouth.	1	
6	Put both hands in the temporal fossa, ask the patient to clench his jaw, and feel a lump on both sides.	1	
7	Ask the patient to keep the mouth slightly open, put a finger on the lower jaw stroke it with a hammer, and watch for upward movement of the jaw.	1	
8	Ask the patient to look upwards with eyes wide open and touch just lateral to the pupil with a cotton wisp and look for a blink on both sides.	1	
B	**Assessment of Professional Behavior**		
1	Addressed the patient appropriately and introduced himself/herself by name	1	
2	Informed patient regarding completion of the procedure and thanked the patient before leaving	1	
III	**Total Marks (Tick)**	10	
	Final Score		
	Global Rating: 1. Poor; 2. Unsatisfactory; 3. Satisfactory; 4. Good; 5. Excellent		
	Observer's comment (based on general observation)		
	Signature of the Observer		

Introduction:

Students will be evaluated for examination of the 5th cranial nerve (Trigeminal nerve). The student needs to understand the clinical technique and interpretation of the findings. The trigeminal nerve has both sensory and motor components. It is also involved in the reflex arc of the Jaw jerk and corneal reflex.

Expected from a student:

- The student should be well apprisedof the use of cotton for sensory examination and a hammer for jaw jerk.
- The student should be acquainted with the proper steps of eliciting the sensory examination and reflexes.
- The student needs to be aware of the expected result and its interpretation.

Clinical application:

- Examining the sensory distribution of trigeminal nerve
- Assessing motor supply of trigeminal nerve
- Elicitation of Jaw jerk and Corneal reflex

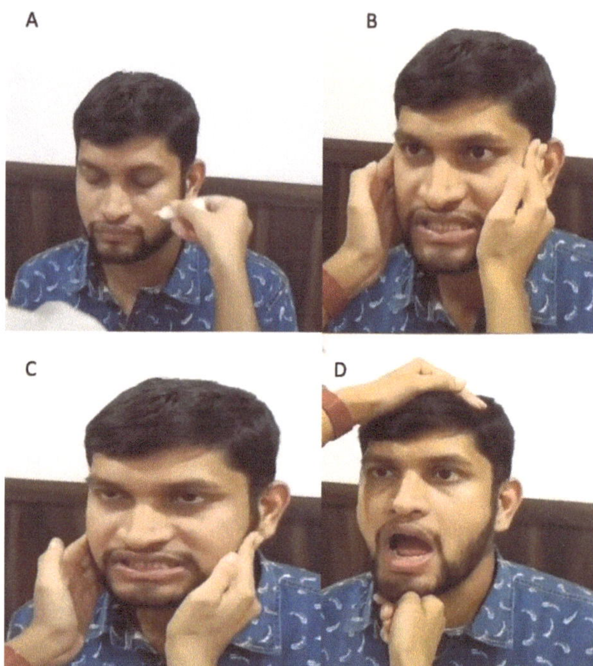

Figure A.e.1 – A: Testing the sensory division of trigeminal nerve (facial sensations); **B:** Palpating the temporalis muscle while the patient is asked to clench teeth; **C:** Palpating the masseter muscle while the patient is asked to clench teeth; **D:**Examining for the pterygoid muscles while the patient is asked to open the mouth against examiner's resistance (Jaw deviates to the paralyzed side)

Trigeminal nerve:

The trigeminal nerve has two divisions. The sensory division had 3 subdivisions: 1) Ophthalmic 2) Maxillary 3) Mandibular, all of which carry sensations from the face. The main sensory and motor nuclei are located in mid-pons. The smaller motor part innervates the muscles of mastication. The proprioceptive component of the trigeminal nerve originates from the mesencephalic nucleus which is also located in the pons.

The sensory part receives sensations from the face (except the angle of the mandible), the anterior part of the scalp, the eye, and the anterior two-thirds of the tongue, teeth, oral cavity, and nasal cavity. The motor part supplies muscles of mastication: masseter, temporal muscles, and pterygoids. The trigeminal nerve is involved in the reflex arc of jaw jerk and corneal reflex.

Procedure:

Sensory examination: Superficial skin sensations are tested on 3 areas of the face,

1. Ophthalmic area
2. Maxillary area
3. Mandibular area

Motor examination: Any wasting of muscles of mastication is inspected by observing the hollowing of the temple (temporal muscles) and flattening of the angle of the jaw (masseter). The examiner must put hands on the anterior part of the tragus on both sides of the face and watch for forward or sideward movement of hands to assess the power of the masseter. The examiner will put hands below the jaw and the patient will be asked to open his mouth wide open to assess the power of pterygoids. The examiner will put hands in the temporal fossa and the patient will be asked to clench his jaw and examiner will look for bulging of the fossa to assess the power of temporal muscles.

Reflexes:

1. **Jaw jerk:** The patient will be asked to keep their mouth slightly open and the examiner will put his finger on the lower lip and gently stroke it with a hammer and look for upward movement of the jaw.
2. **Corneal reflex:** The patient will be asked to look upwards and keep eyes wide open. Later, a cotton wisp will be touched gently just lateral to the pupil and the examiner will look for the blink of the eyes in both eyes.

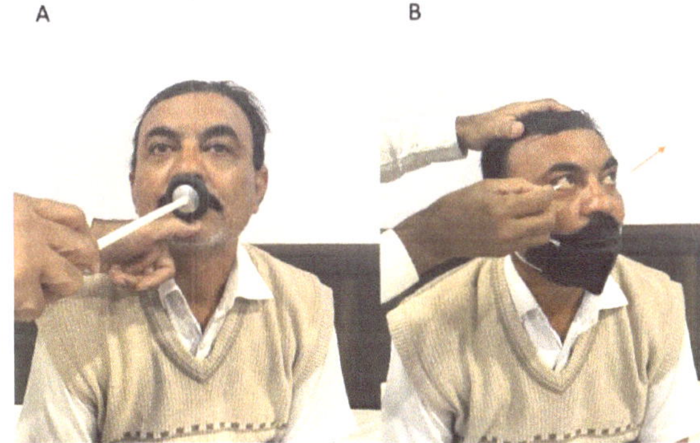

Figure A.e.2 – A: Method of eliciting the Jaw Jerk; **B:** Method of eliciting the corneal reflex (afferent nerve-5th nerve and efferent nerve – 7th nerve)

Abnormalities on examination:

- Total loss of sensation in the whole distribution of nerve: Tumours of the base of the skull, large neurofibromata 5th and 7th nerves.
- Total sensory loss over one or more of the main divisions: Herpes zoster, acoustic neuroma, carotid aneurysm.
- Dissociative sensory loss: syringomyelia, syringobulbia.
- Pain and temperature loss: Lateral medullary lesion, Pontine lesion.
- Wasting of muscles of mastication: Motor neuron disease, compression of the motor root by tumor (unilateral), muscular dystrophy.
- Minimal or absent jaw jerk: Normal variant.
- Exaggerated jaw jerk: pseudobulbar palsy, motor neuron disease, multiple sclerosis

f. Seventh Cranial nerve – Facial nerve

Table A.f.1: Checklist

Type of Station: Examination of the 7th cranial nerve in the patient

Domain: Cognitive, Psychomotor, Affective.

Communication Time: 1 minute

Marks: 10

Sr no	Steps	Marks	R. No
I	**Checklist**		
1	Stands on the right of the patient, Makes the subject comfortable, Explains the procedure in the local language	1	
2	Checks facial symmetry like deviation of angle of mouth, and loss of nasolabial fold.	1	
3	Examines muscles of facial expression like frontalis, orbicularis oculi, buccinators, orbicularis oris, platysma	2	
4	Checks for bells phenomenon	1	
5	Taste sensation on anterior 2/3 of tongue	2	
6	Check corneal reflex	1	
II	**Assessment of professional behavior**		
1	Addressed the patient appropriately and introduced himself/herself by name	1	
2	Informed patient regarding completion of the procedure and thanked the patient before leaving	1	
III	**Total Marks (Tick)**	10	
	Final Score		
	Global Rating: 1. Poor; 2. Unsatisfactory; 3. Satisfactory; 4. Good; 5. Excellent		
	Observer's comment (based on general observation)		
	Signature of the Observer		

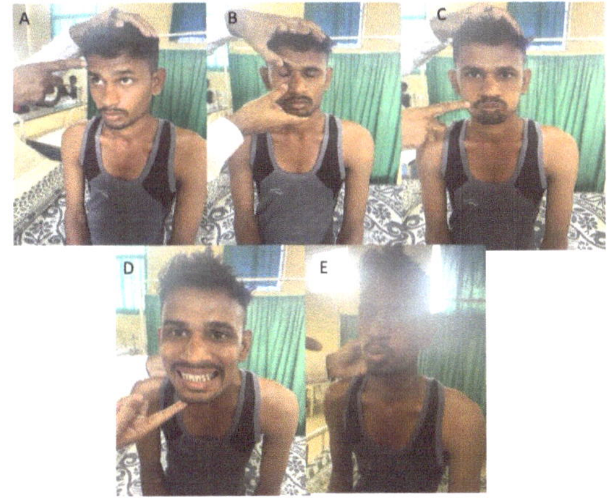

Figure A.f.1 – A: Testing for the frontal belly of occipitofrontal muscle; **B:** Testing for orbicularis oculi; **C:** Testing for buccinators muscle; **D:** testing for platysma muscle; **E:** Testing for orbicularis oris.

Introduction:

Students will be evaluated for examination of facial nerve. The student needs to understand the clinical technique and interpretation of the clinical findings. The facial nerve is the 7th cranial nerve with motor, sensory, and parasympathetic components.

Expected from a student:

- The student should be well apprised with the area supplied by the facial nerve and the clinal techniques to assess its function.
- The student should be acquainted with the proper steps of eliciting the required reflexes for the assessment of facial nerve.
- The student needs to be aware of the expected result and its interpretation.

Clinical application:

- Examination of facial nerve
- To differentiate UMN from LMN lesion

Notes:

Facial Nerve:

The facial nerve has motor, sensory, and parasympathetic components. The upper half of the face has a bilateral innervation by the facial nerve, whereas the lower half of the face has a unilateral innervation.

Figure A.f.2 – Course of the facial nerve

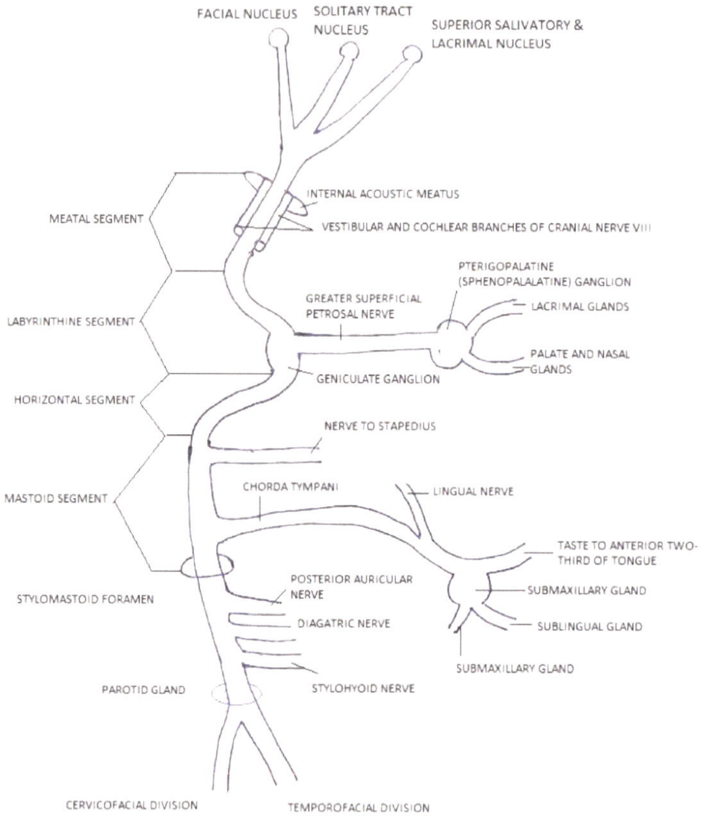

Table A.f.2: Examination of Facial Nerve

Inspection:	1. Observe the face for any asymmetry which may be related to paresis of facial muscles 2. Check for atrophy	
Motor function:	1. Wrinkle the forehead	Frontal belly of Occipito-frontalis
	2. Close the eyes as tightly as possible while trying to open eyelid with fingers.	Orbicularis Occuli
	3. Ask patient to show his teeth or smile	Orbicularis Oris
	4. To blow out the cheeks and tap each cheek with finger	Buccinator
	5. Ask patient to clench his teeth and simultaneously depress mouth	Platysma
Sensory system	Taste sensation of anterior 2/3 of tongue	
Parasympathetic	Lacrimation is tested by schirmers test	
Reflexes	1. Conjunctival reflex 2. Corneal reflex 3. Stapedial reflex	

Table A.f.3: Common causes of facial nerve palsy

Unilateral	Bilateral
UMN	
Usually Vascular • Cerebral tumor • Multiple sclerosis	Often vascular (multi-infarct dementia) • Motor Neuron Disease
LMN	
• Bell's palsy • Parotid tumor • Head injuries • Skull base tumor • Diabetes • Hypertension	• Guillain-Barre' syndrome • Sarcoidosis-Uveoparotid fever • Leprosy • Leukemia/Lymphoma • Ramsey hunt syndrome (Herpes zoster)

Differences between UMN and LMN types of facial nerve palsy:

Only the lower part of the face is involved in UMN palsy on the contralateral side.

In LMN facial palsy, the unilateral whole face is involved and there is the presence of hyperacusis and loss of taste sensation in the anterior 2/3rd of the tongue because of palsy of the nerve to stapedius and chorda tympany.

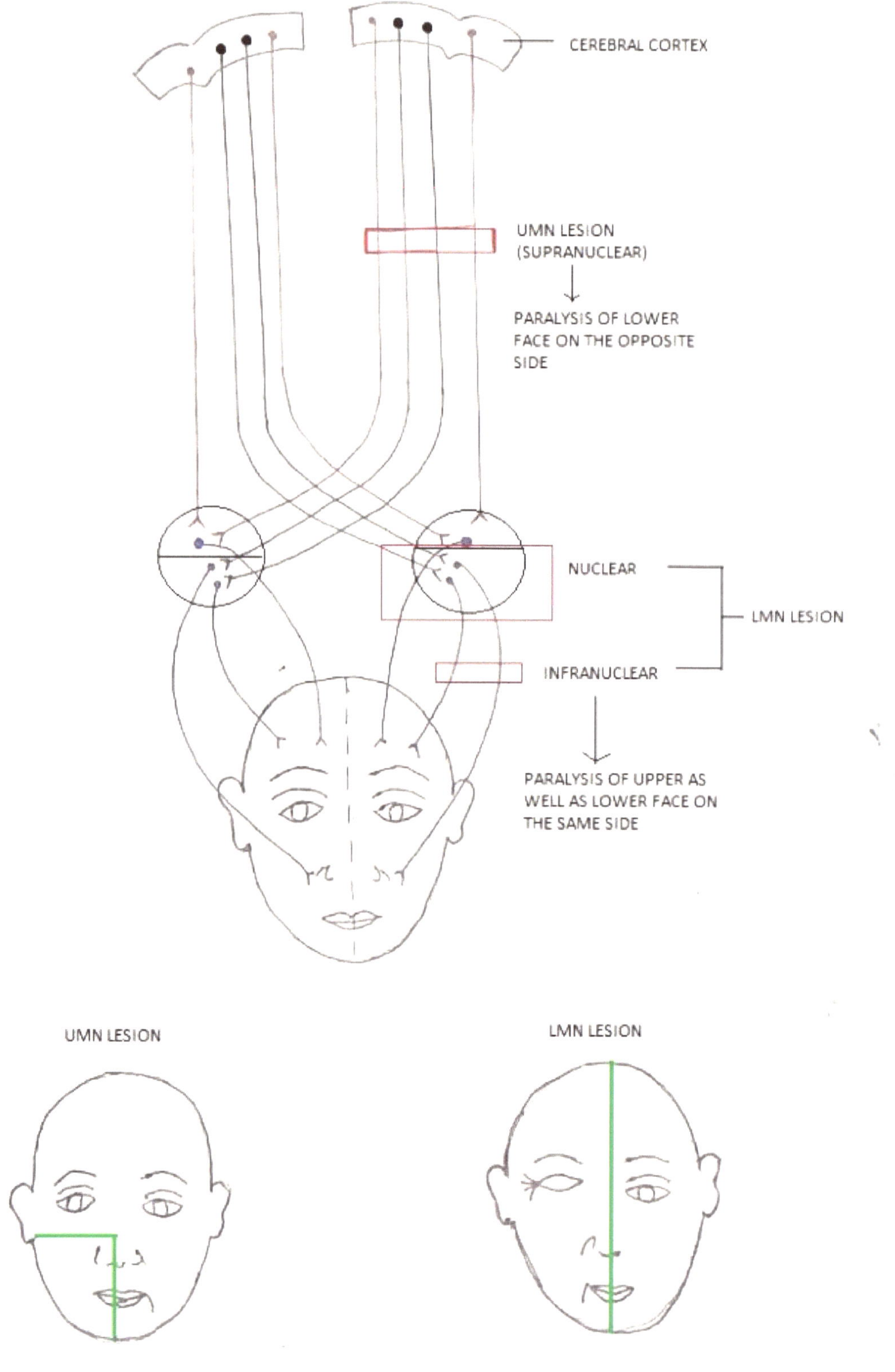

Figure A.f.3: Showing Features of UMN and LMN Facial Nerve Palsy.

g. Ninth and Tenth Cranial nerves (Glossopharyngeal and Vagus nerve)

Table A.g.1: Checklist

Type of Station: Examination of the 9 and 10th cranial nerve in the patient

Domain: Cognitive, Psychomotor, Affective.

Communication Time: 1 minute
Marks: 10

Sr. no	Steps	Marks	Roll no.
I	**Checklist**		
1	Stands in front of the subject, Makes the subject comfortable in a sitting position and explains the procedure.	1	
2	Noticed for the pitch and quality of voice and his/her cough	1	
3	Looked for any difficulty in swallowing saliva and nasal regurgitation	1	
4	Asked the patient to say "AHH" while in the expiration	1	
5	Looked for the movement of the palate and uvula	2	
6	Summarised the findings	2	
II	**Assessment of professional behavior**		
1	Addressed the patient appropriately and introduced himself/herself by name	1	
2	Informed patient regarding completion of the procedure and thanked the patient before leaving	1	
III	**Total Marks (Tick)**	**10**	
	Final Score		
	Global rating: 1. Poor; 2. Unsatisfactory; 3.satisfactory; 4. Good; 5. Excellent		
	Observer's comment (based on general observation)		
	Signature of the Observer		

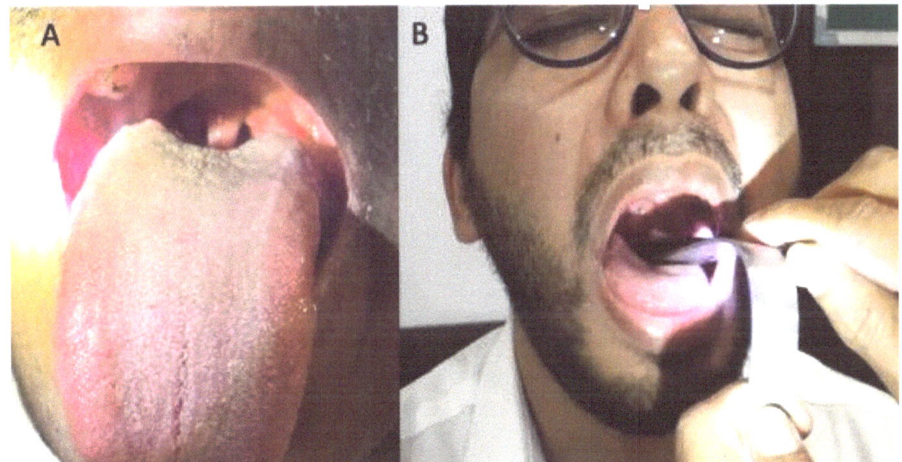

Figure A.g.1 A: Testing for the central position of the uvula , **B:** Testing for Gag reflex (afferent nerve-9th nerve and efferent nerve-10th nerve)

Introduction

The glossopharyngeal nerve (IXth) carries motor, sensory,andparasympatheticfibers.

The motor fibers originate from the nucleus ambiguous and supply the stylopharyngeus muscle and (with the vagus nerve) muscles of the pharynx.

It also carries taste sensations from the posterior third of the tongue and the pharynx, and sensations from the posterior third of the tongue, tonsils, palatal arch, soft palate, nasopharynx, and tragus of the ear.

The vagus nerve (Xth nerve) carries motor, sensory, and parasympathetic nervefibers. The dorsal motor nucleus of the vagus gives rise to preganglionic parasympathetic fibers that innervate the pharynx, respiratory, and gastrointestinal systems. Through the vagus, the nucleus ambiguoussupplies all of the striated musculature of the soft palate, pharynx,and larynx except the tensor velipalatine

What is expected from the student

- The student should be well apprised with the integrity of the reflex arc for the gag reflex
- The student should be acquainted with the proper steps for electing the reflex
- The student needs to be aware of the expected result and its interpretation.

Clinical Application

The patient is asked to open their mouth and say "Aah". In a normal person, both palatal arches rise simultaneously and the uvula goes up. In vagus nerve palsy, the palatal arch lags on the affected side and the uvula is shifted to the opposite side. (This test is only for the vagus nerve)

Test for both 9th and 10th [gag reflex – afferent 9th and efferent 10th]: Patient is asked to open the mouth and the roof of the palate is touched by a soft cotton applicator and movement of the uvula is seen.

Interpretation: normal person, uvula goes up. The abnormal response is uvula shifted to the opposite side.

h. Eleventh Cranial Nerve (The Accessory Nerve)

Table A.h.1: Checklist

Procedural station

Eliciting the examination of the 11th cranial nerve

Domain: Cognitive, Psychomotor, Affective.

Communication Time: 1 minute   Marks-10

Sr. no	Steps	Marks	R.no
I	**Checklist**		
1	Stands in front of the subject, Makes the subject comfortable in a sitting position and explains the procedure.	1	
2	Inspect for sternocleidomastoid muscle by turning the head to the opposite side.	1	
3	Inspect the trapezius muscle atrophy by looking for depression of shoulder contour or shagging and flattening of the trapezius ridge	1	
4	Ask the patient to turn their head to each side against resistance	2	
5	Ask the patient to shrug their shoulders against resistance	2	
6	Examined both sides	1	
II	**Assessment of Professional Behavior**		
1	Addressed the patient appropriately and introduced himself/herself by name	1	
2	Informed patient regarding completion of the procedure and thanked the patient before leaving	1	
III	**Total Marks (Tick)**	10	
	FINAL SCORE		
	Global Rating: 1. Poor; 2. Unsatisfactory; 3. Satisfactory; 4. Good; 5. Excellent		
	Observer's comment (based on general observation)		
	Signature of the Observer		

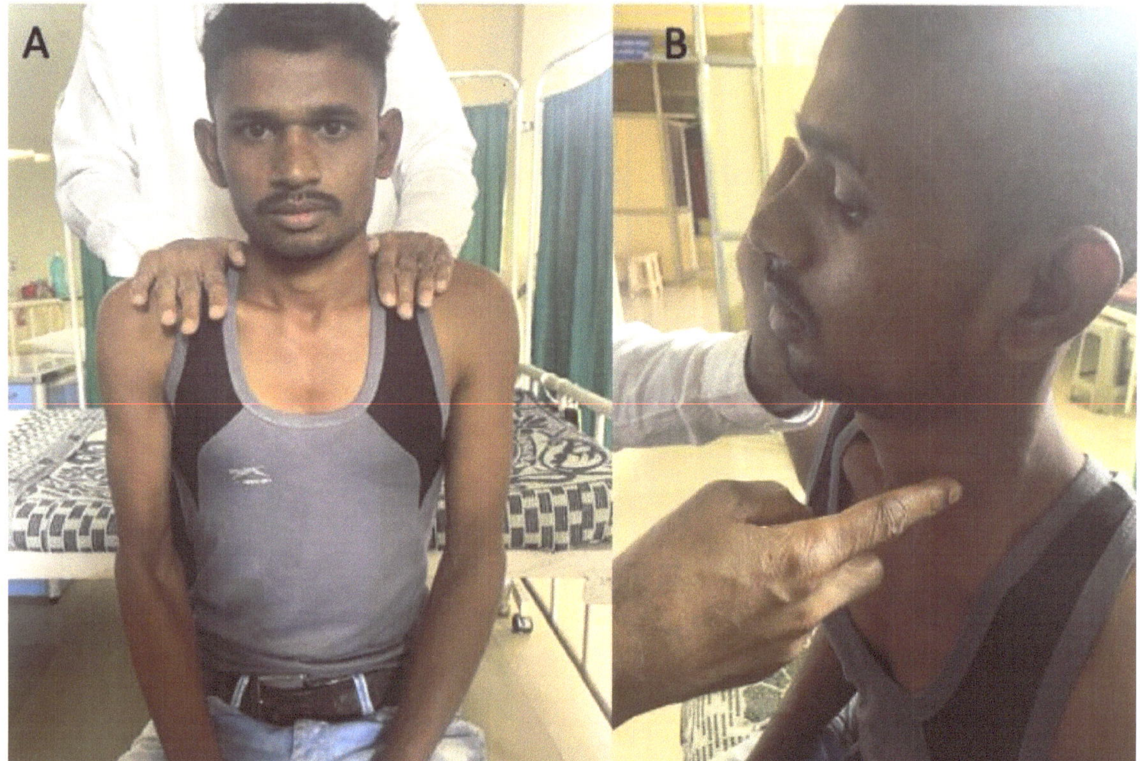

Figure A.h.1 – A: Testing for the function of the spinal accessory nerve (Power of the trapezius muscle is assessed by asking the patient to shrug the shoulder against resistance); **B:** Testing for the contraction of the sternocleidomastoid muscle (patient is asked to move his head laterally against resistance)

Introduction:

Students will be evaluated for **eliciting the examination of 11ᵗʰcranialnerve.** The student needs to understand the clinical technique and interpretation of the examination of the 11ᵗʰ cranial nerve. The 11ᵗʰ nerve supplies the sternocleidomastoid and trapezius muscle.

Expected from a student:

- The student should be able to detect wasting and weakness, unilateral or bilateral of, the muscles.

Clinical application:

- To inspect sternocleidomastoid and trapezius muscle wasting.
- To detect wasting, weakness, involuntary movement, and myotonia
- To examine voluntary muscle control

Notes:

The spinal root originates from the spinal nucleus located in the spinal grey column (accessory nucleus) and descends up to the C5 spinal segment. The cranial part arises from the caudal part of the nucleus ambigus. The cranial and spinal roots join and exit through the jugular foramen. The cranial part joins the Xᵗʰ(vagus) nerve and supplies the larynx and pharynx. The spinal part supplies the sternocleidomastoid and trapezius muscles.

Method of examination: On inspection, severe trapezius weakness is suspected if the head falls forward and sternomastoid weakness if it falls backward.

Sternomastoid:

Place one hand against the right side of the patient's face and ask him to turn his head against it. The left sternomastoid will stand out clearly. Repeat this in the opposite direction and compare the two sides for bulk and strength.

Trapezius:

Stand behind the patient and compare the line and curve of the trapezii and the position of the scapulae. Asking the patient to raise his shoulder against the resistance.

Common lesions of theAccessory nerve:

1. **Bilateral**

- Nuclear 11th nerve – Motor neuron disease, spinal muscular atrophy, poliomyelitis
- Nerve – Polyneuropathy or mononeuropathy
- Muscle – Polymyositis, dermatomyositis, myasthenia gravis, myotonic dystrophy, oculopharyngeal muscular dystrophy

2. **Unilateral**

- Nucleus – Poliomyelitis, syringobulbia
- Nerve – Tumors at jugular foramen level, bony abnormalities of the base of the skull, trauma to the neck or base of the skull, compression to the nerve with enlarged cervical lymph nodes.

i. Twelfth Cranial Nerve (Hypoglossal nerve)

Table A.i.1: Checklist

Procedural station

Eliciting the examination of the 12th cranial nerve

Domain: Cognitive, Psychomotor, Affective.

Communication Time: 1 minute   Marks-10

Sr. no	Steps	Marks	R.no
I	**Checklist**		
1	Stands on the front of the subject made the subject comfortable in a sitting position and explained the procedure.	1	
2	Inspect tongue while relaxed in mouth	1	
3	Use pen light for inspection	1	
4	Tell them to stick out their tongue	1	
5	Tell to move the tongue from side to side	2	
6	Test power by resisting tongue pressed into cheek	2	
II	**Assessment of Professional Behavior**		
1	Addressed the patient appropriately and introduced himself/herself by name	1	
2	Informed patient regarding completion of the procedure and thanked the patient before leaving	1	
III	**Total Marks (Tick)**	10	
	Final Score		
	Global Rating: 1. Poor; 2. Unsatisfactory; 3. Satisfactory; 4. Good; 5. Excellent		
	Observer's comment (based on general observation)		
	Signature of the Observer		

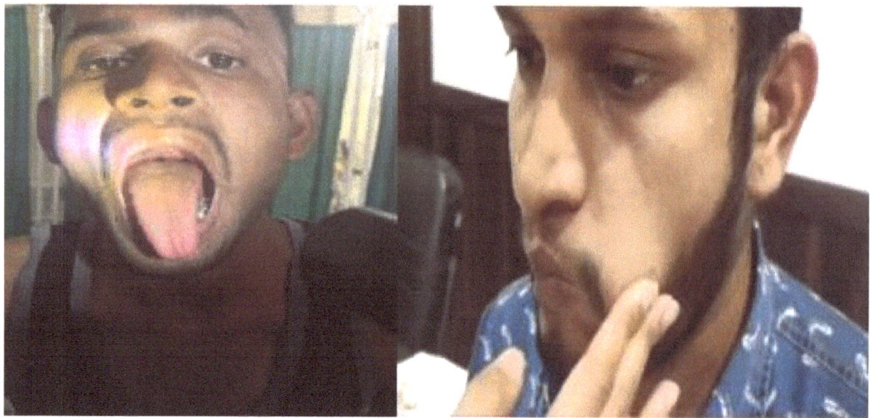

Figure A.i.1: Testing for hyoglossus muscle (Patient is asked to protrude the tongue)

Introduction:

Students will be evaluated for **eliciting the examination of the 12th cranial nerve.** The student needs to understand the clinical technique and interpretation of the examination of the 12th cranial nerve. The 12th nerve controls movements of the tongue, hyoid, and larynx during and after deglutition.

Expected from a student:

- The student should be able to inspect the surface of the tongue
- The student should be able to detect wasting, weakness, and involuntary movements
- The student should be able to examine voluntary muscle control

Clinical application:

- To inspect the surface of the tongue.
- To detect wasting, weakness, involuntary movement, and myotonia
- To examine voluntary muscle control

The hypoglossal nerve supplies all the intrinsic (longitudinal, transverse, and vertical muscles) and extrinsic muscles (hypoglossus, styloglossus, gengioglossus, and geniohyoid muscles) of the tongue except palatoglossus.

Method of examination:

Ask the patient to open his mouth and protrude the tongue in the midline. The surface, size, shape, and position of the tongue are inspected. Note any difficulty in performing the movement, any deviation from the midline, and any involuntary movements, or fasciculations.

Common lesions of the hypoglossal nerve

Lower neuron motor lesions

1) Unilateral

- Syringomyelia
- Poliomyelitis
- Tumors at or near the jugular foramen
- Angiomas of the brainstem
- Trauma
- Tumors or glandular enlargement high in the neck
- Early motor neuron disease

2) Bilateral

- Progressive bulbar palsy
- Syringomyelia
- Foramen magnum anomalies (occasionally)

Upper motor neuron lesions

1. Unilateral

- Profound hemiplegia

2. Bilateral

- Bilateral vascular accidents producing pseudobulbar palsy, amyotrophic

B. Deep and Superficial Tendon Reflexes

Deep Tendon Reflexes:

a. Ankle Jerk/Reflex
Table B.a.1: Checklist
Type of Station: Procedural station
Eliciting the ankle reflex in the patient
Domain: Cognitive, Psychomotor, Affective.
Communication Time: 1 minute   Marks-10

Sr. no	Steps	Marks	Roll.no
I	**Checklist**		
1	Stands on the right side of the subject and makes the subject comfortable in lying down position and explains the procedure.	1	
2	Exposes the leg of the subject properly up to the knee	1	
3	Flexes the knee and dorsiflexes the ankle with slight inversion of the foot	1	
4	Palpate the Achilles Tendon	1	
5	Tap the Achilles Tendon of the patient with the hammer having movement at the wrist joint	1	
6	Observe for the contraction of the gastrocnemius muscle	1	
7	Look for the Jendrassik maneuver in case of an absent reflex	1	
8	Repeat the procedure in the other limb as well	1	
II	**Assessment of Professional Behavior**		
1	Addressed the patient appropriately and introduced himself/herself by name	1	
2	Informed patient regarding completion of the procedure and thanked the patient before leaving	1	
III	**Total Marks (Tick)**	10	
	Final Score		
	Global Rating: 1. Poor; 2. Unsatisfactory; 3. Satisfactory; 4. Good; 5. Excellent		
	Observer's Comment (based on general observation)		
	Signature of the Observer		

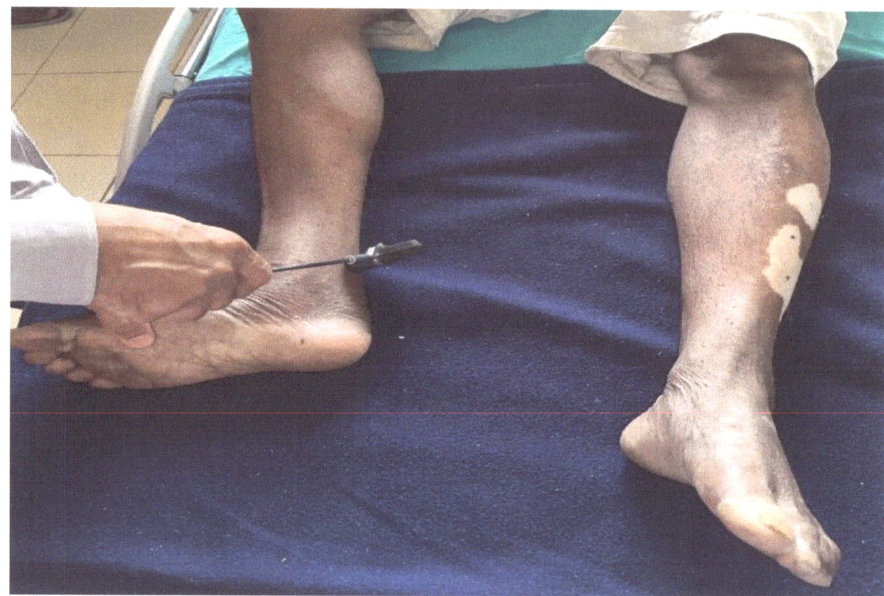

Figure B.a.1: Demonstrating ankle reflex

Introduction:

Students will be evaluated for demonstration of Ankle Jerk with the help of a knee hammer. The student needs to understand the clinical technique and interpretation of the Ankle Jerk. The ankle jerk reflex, also known as the Achilles reflex, occurs when the Achilles tendon is tapped while the foot is dorsiflexed and slight inversion. It is a monosynaptic spinal segmental reflex. The root value is S1-S2.

Expected from a student:

- The student should be well apprised of the use of a hammer such as movement at the wrist and not at the elbow or shoulder.
- The student should be acquainted with the proper steps of eliciting the reflex.
- The student needs to be aware of the expected result and its interpretation.

Clinical application:

- Eliciting the Ankle Jerk
- Root Value of the reflex
- Grading of reflexes:

  0 = absent
  1 = present but diminished
  2 =normoactive
  3 = exaggerated
  4 = clonus

Notes:

Ankle Jerk/Reflex

The ankle jerk/reflex occurs when the Achilles tendon is tapped while the foot is dorsiflexed. It tests the function of the gastrocnemius muscle and the nerve that supplies it. **A positive result would be the jerking of the foot towards its plantar surface**

Root Value: S1,S2 spinal segment of the spinal cord

Procedure: Legs should be exposed up to the knee with a relaxed Ankle joint. The knee is flexed and supports the lateral aspect of the foot on the couch with slight dorsiflexion and inversion to put some tension in the Achilles tendon. A small strike is given on the Achilles tendon using a rubber hammer with movement on the wrist joint to elicit the response in the form of contraction of the gastrocnemius muscle. If the practitioner is not able to elicit a response, a Jendrassik maneuver can be tried by having the patient make a fist on each hand, or clinching of the teeth. Students must remember that striking on tendons should be done at the time of clinching of teeth or making of a fist, not before that. A positive response is marked by a brisk plantar flexion of the foot.

Jendrassik maneuver: The briskness of deep tendon reflexes sometimes can only be elicited in normal individuals by applying reinforcement known as the Jendrassik maneuver. This happens due to anterior horn cell excitability. The upper limb reflexes may be reinforced by voluntary teeth-clenching and the Achilles reflex by hooking the flexed fingers of the two hands together and attempting to pull them apart. Reinforcement is greatest for only a fraction of a second after the onset of contraction, so the examiner must explain the request beforehand and test the reflex as soon as the patient starts.

Causes of absent Ankle Jerk:

- Disk herniations at the L5-S1 level.
- Peripheral neuropathy
- Cauda equina syndrome

It is classically delayed in hypothyroidism, known as **Hung up reflex**

Exaggerated ankle reflex: UMN paralysis

b. Knee Jerk/Reflex

Table B.b.1: Checklist

Type of Station: Procedural station

Eliciting the Knee Reflex

Domain: Cognitive, Psychomotor, Affective.

Communication Time: 1 minute

Marks-10

Sr. no	Steps	Marks	Roll.no
I	**Checklist**		
1	Stands on the right side of the subject and makes the subject comfortable in lying down position and explains the procedure.	1	
2	Exposes the leg of the subject properly up to the thigh	1	
3	Flexes the knee in such a way so that the heel of the foot only touches the couch, or With the patient supine, pass your hand under the knee to be tested so that it supports the relaxed leg with the knee flexed at a little less than 90°.	1	
4	Palpate the patellar Tendon above the tibial tuberosity	1	
5	Tap the patellar Tendon with the hammer having movement at the wrist joint	1	
6	Observe The Contraction of the quadriceps muscle	1	
7	Look for the Jendrassik maneuver in case of an absent reflex	1	
8	Repeat the procedure in the other limb as well	1	
II	**Assessment of Professional Behavior**		
1	Addressed the patient appropriately and introduced himself/herself by name	1	
2	Informed patient regarding completion of the procedure and thanked the patient before leaving	1	
III	**Total Marks (Tick)**	10	
	Final Score		
	Global Rating: 1. Poor; 2. Unsatisfactory; 3. Satisfactory; 4. Good; 5. Excellent		
	Observer's Comment (based on general observation)		
	Signature of the Observer		

Introduction:

Students will be evaluated for demonstration of Knee Jerk with the help of a knee hammer. The student needs to understand the clinical technique of eliciting the reflex and interpretation of the same. The root value of the **patellar reflex** or **knee-jerk** is the L2, L3, and L4 segments of the spinal cord.After the tap of a hammer, the leg is normally extended once due to contraction of the quadriceps muscle and comes to rest

Expected from a student:

- Method of eliciting the reflex
- The student should be aware of the required instrument to elicit the knee jerk.
- The student should be well apprised of the handling of the instruments.
- The student should be acquainted with the proper steps of eliciting the knee jerk.
- The student needs to be aware of the expected result and its interpretation.

Clinical application:

- Eliciting the knee jerk
- Should know causes of exaggerated/diminished/absent knee-jerk
- Root value of the knee-jerk

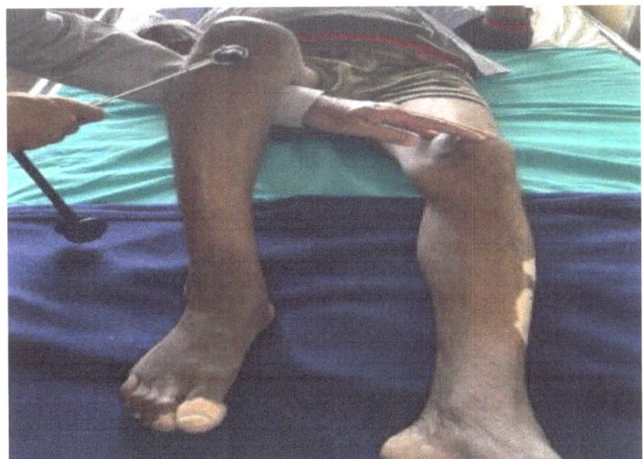

Figure B.b.1: Eliciting Knee Reflex

Knee reflex – Procedure: The knee should be flexed in such a way so that the heel of the foot slightly touches the couch, while the patient is supine, pass your hand under the knee to be tested so that it supports the relaxed leg with the knee flexed at a little less than 90° then striking of the patellar tendon with a reflex hammer just below the patella stretches the muscle spindle in the quadriceps muscle leading to visible contraction of quadriceps muscles. The patellar reflex is a clinical and classic example of the monosynaptic reflex arc. Always use the maneuver to ensure valid reflex test before saying absent.

Root value – L 2,3,4

Causes of exaggerated knee reflex:

- UMN paralysis, Anxiety, hyperthyroidism

Causes of absent knee jerk:

- LMN lesion
- Patient keeping the joint too tight

Pendular jerk

- Multiple oscillations (2.5 times) of the leg following the tap – - – cerebellar diseases.

c. Biceps Jerk/Reflex

Table B.c.1: Checklist

Type of Station: Procedural station

Eliciting the biceps reflex in the patient

Domain: Cognitive, Psychomotor, Affective.

Communication Time: 1 minute

Marks-10

Sr. no	Steps	Marks	Roll.no
I	**Checklist**		
1	Stands on the right side of the subject and makes the subject comfortable in lying down position and explains the procedure.	1	
2	Exposes the arm of the subject properly up to the shoulder	1	
3	Flexes the elbow and forearm kept on the abdomen in a neutral position	1	
4	Palpate and put the index finger on the biceps Tendon	1	
5	Tap the biceps Tendon of the patient with the hammer having movement at the wrist joint	1	
6	Observes for the contraction of the biceps muscle	1	
7	Look for the Jendrassik maneuver in case of an absent reflex	1	
8	Repeat the procedure in the other limb as well	1	
II	**Assessment of Professional Behaviour**		
1	Addressed the patient appropriately and Introduced himself/herself by name	1	
2	Informed patient regarding completion of the procedure and Thanked the patient before leaving	1	
III	**Total Marks (Tick)**	10	
	Final Score		
	Global Rating: 1. Poor; 2. Unsatisfactory; 3. Satisfactory; 4. Good; 5. Excellent		
	Observer's Comment (based on general observation):		
	Signature of the Observer		

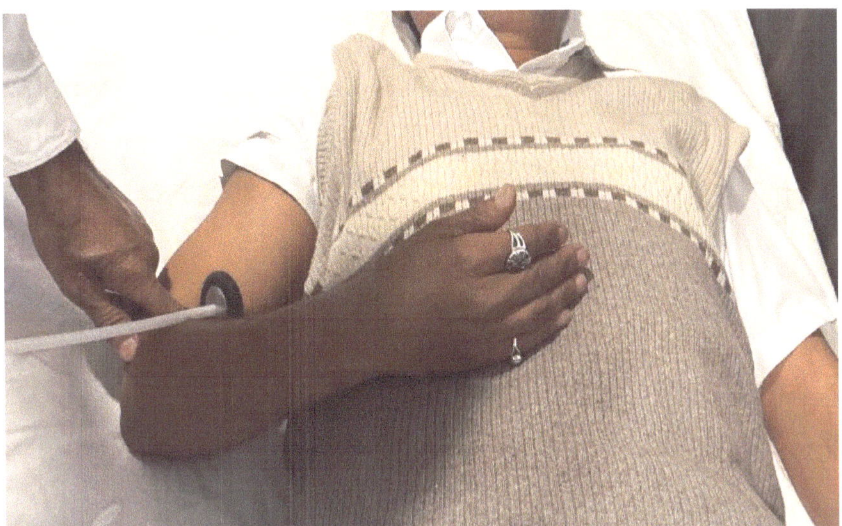

Figure B.c.1: Demonstrating the Biceps Reflex

Introduction:

Students will be evaluated for demonstration of Biceps Jerk with the help of a hammer. The student needs to understand the clinical technique and interpretation of the Biceps Jerk. It is elicited when the Biceps tendon is tapped while the arm is semiflexed at the elbow and the forearm rests on the abdomen in a neutral position, while the patient is lying down in a supine position and relaxed. The biceps tendon should not be hammered directly but on the indexed figure kept on it. It is a type of stretch reflex that tests the function of the biceps muscle and the nerve that supplies it. These are monosynaptic spinal segmental reflexes.

Expected from a student:

- The student should be well apprised of the use of a hammer such as movement at the wrist and not at the elbow or shoulder.
- The student should be acquainted with the proper steps of eliciting the reflex.
- The student needs to be aware of the expected result and its interpretation.

Clinical application:

- Eliciting the biceps Jerk
- Root Value of the reflex
- Inversion of reflexes

Notes:

Root Value: C5,6 spinal cord segment

Procedure: The patient's elbow is flexed with an aspect to the forearm so that it makes a 90-degree angle with it in semi-pronation while resting on the abdomen/chest. Use the index finger to localize the biceps tendon, and strike the tendon with firmness using a patellar hammer. Then the contraction of the biceps muscle is observed. If there is no contraction then the Jendrassik maneuver should be tried.

Absent reflex: LMN paralysis

Exaggerated reflex: UMN paralysis

Inversion of reflex: With lesions at the level of C5 (cervical myelopathy) the biceps jerk may be absent along with a brisk flexion of the fingers present instead. This is known as inversion of the reflex and suggests hyper excitability of anterior horn cells below the affected level.

d. Triceps Jerk/Reflex

Table B.d.1: Checklist

Type of Station: Eliciting the biceps reflex in the patient
Domain: Cognitive, Psychomotor, Affective.
Communication Time: 1 minute   Marks-10

Sr. no	Steps	Marks	Roll.no
I	**Checklist**		
1	Stands on the right side of the subject and makes the subject comfortable in lying down position and explains the procedure.	1	
2	Exposes the arm of the subject properly up to the shoulder	1	
3	Flexes the elbow and forearm kept on the abdomen in a neutral position	1	
4	Palpate the Triceps Tendon	1	
5	Tap the Triceps Tendon of the patient with the hammer having movement at the wrist joint	1	
6	Observe for the contraction of the Triceps muscle	1	
7	Look for the Jendrassik maneuver in case of an absent reflex	1	
8	Repeat the procedure in the other limb as well	1	
II	**Assessment of Professional Behavior**		
1	Addressed the patient appropriately and introduced himself/herself by name	1	
2	Informed patient regarding completion of the procedure and thanked the patient before leaving	1	
III	**Total Marks (Tick)**	10	
	Final Score		
	Global Rating: 1. Poor; 2. Unsatisfactory; 3. Satisfactory; 4. Good; 5. Excellent		
	Observer's Comment (based on general observation)		
	Signature of the Observer		

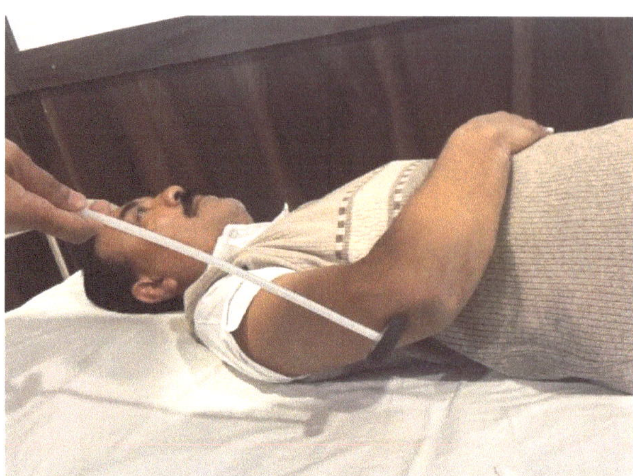

Figure B.d.1: Demonstrating triceps reflex

Introduction:

Students will be evaluated for demonstration of Triceps Jerk with the help of a hammer. The student needs to understand the clinical technique and interpretation of the Triceps Jerk. It is elicited when the Triceps tendon is tapped while the arm is semi-flexed at the elbow and the forearm rests on the abdomen in a neutral position, while the patient is lying down in a supine position and relaxed. These are monosynaptic spinal segmental reflexes.

Expected from a student:

- The student should be well apprised of the use of a hammer such as movement at the wrist and not at the elbow or shoulder.
- The student should be acquainted with the proper steps of eliciting the reflex.
- The student needs to be aware of the expected result and its interpretation.

Clinical application:

- Eliciting the Jerk
- Root Value of the reflex
- Grading of reflexes

Notes:

Root Value: This reflex is mediated by the C6,7 spinal segment of the spinal cord

Procedure: Flex the patient's elbow with the forearm resting across the chest or on the abdomen. Tap the triceps tendon just above the olecranon. The triceps contracts. The Jendrassik maneuver can be tried in case there is no visible contraction.

Absent Triceps Jerk: AIDP, CIDP, Cervical myelopathy at C7 level, brachial plexopathy, LMN motor neuron disease.

Exaggerated Triceps reflex: UMN paralysis, C5 myelopathy, High cervical cord lesion, Hemiplegia, Anxiety.

e. Supinator Jerk/Reflex

Table B.e.1: Checklist

Type of Station: Procedural station
Eliciting the Supinator reflex in the patient
Domain: Cognitive, Psychomotor, Affective.
Communication Time: 1 minute   Marks-10

Sr. no	Steps	Marks	Roll.no
I	**Checklist**		
1	Stands on the right side of the subject and makes the subject comfortable in lying down position and explains the procedure.	1	
2	Exposes the forearm of the subject properly up to the elbow	1	
3	Flexes the elbow and forearm kept in a semi-prone position on the abdomen in a neutral position	1	
4	Palpate the supinator tendon 2-3 cm below the styloid process of the radius bone	1	
5	Tap the supinator Tendon of the patient with the hammer having movement at the wrist joint	1	
6	Observes for the contraction of the brachioradialis muscle	1	
7	Look for the Jendrassik maneuver in case of an absent reflex	1	
8	Repeat the procedure in the other limb as well	1	
II	**Assessment of Professional Behavior**		
1	Addressed the patient appropriately and introduced himself/herself by name	1	
2	Informed patient regarding completion of the procedure and thanked the patient before leaving	1	
III	**Total Marks (Tick)**	10	
	Final Score		
	Global Rating: 1. Poor; 2. Unsatisfactory; 3. Satisfactory; 4. Good; 5. Excellent		
	Observer's Comment (based on general observation):		
	Signature of the Observer		

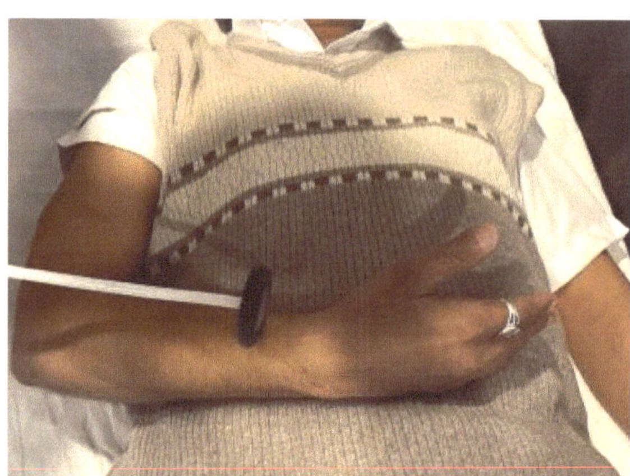

Figure B.e.1: Demonstrating Supinator Reflex

Introduction:

Students will be evaluated for demonstration of Supinator Jerk with the help of a hammer. The student needs to understand the clinical technique and interpretation of the Supinator Jerk. It is elicited when the supinator tendon is tapped while the arm is semiflexed and semi proned at the elbow and the forearm rests on the abdomen in a neutral position, while the patient is lying down in a supine position and relaxed. The supinator tendon should be tapped 2-3 cm below the styloid process of the radius bone. It is a type of stretch reflex that tests the function of the biceps muscle and the nerve that supplies it. These are monosynaptic spinal segmental reflexes.

Expected from a student:

- The student should be well apprised of the use of a hammer such as movement at the wrist and not at the elbow or shoulder.
- The student should be acquainted with the proper steps of eliciting the reflex.
- The student needs to be aware of the expected result and its interpretation

Root Value: This reflex is mediated by the C5,6 spinal segment of the spinal cord

Absent Jerk: LMN

Exaggerated reflex: UMN paralysis

Inversion of reflex: With mid-cervical lesions at the level of C5 (cervical myelopathy) the

supinator jerks may be absent but brisk flexion of the fingers may occur instead.

Superficial reflexes:

f. Planter reflex/Babinski reflex

Table B.f.1: Checklist
Type of Station: Eliciting the planter reflex in the patient
Domain: Cognitive, Psychomotor, Affective.
Communication Time: 1 minute   Marks-10

Sr. no	Steps	Marks	Roll.no
I	**Checklist**		
1.	Stands on the right side of the subject and makes subject comfortable in lying down position and explained the procedure.	1	
2.	Stimulation of the lateral plantar aspect of the foot with blunt end of patellar hammer or key from the heel to the toes, and across the metatarsal pads to the base of the big toe. Avoid touching ball of big toe.	1	
3.	Watch for the movement of big toe	1	
4.	Watch for other response like, Fanning of other toes, Dorsiflexion at ankle, Flexion at knee and Contraction of tensor fascia lata and flexion and hip joint	1	
5.	Looked for Chaddock (stimulating under lateral malleolus),	1	
6.	Looked for Gordon (squeezing calf),	1	
7.	Look for Oppenheim (applying pressure to the medial side of the tibia),	1	
8.	Repeat the procedure in other limb as well	1	
II	**Assessment of Professional Behavior**		
1	Addressed patient appropriately and introduced himself/herself by name	1	
2	Informed patient regarding completion of the procedure and thanked the patient before leaving	1	
III	**Total Marks (Tick)**	10	
	Final Score		
	Global Rating: 1. Poor; 2. Unsatisfactory; 3. Satisfactory; 4. Good; 5. Excellent		
	Observer's Comment (based on general observation)		
	Signature of the Observer		

The Babinski reflex was described by the neurologist Joseph Babinski in 1899.

The Babinski reflex tests the integrity of the corticospinal tract,Damage anywhere along this tract can result in the presence of a positive Babinski sign.

The normal response is plantar flexion of the great toe.

Normally the corticospinal tract keeps the ascending sensory stimulation from spreading to other nerve roots. When the corticospinal tract/pyramidal tract is damaged, nociceptive input spreads beyond S1 anterior horn cells leading to L4/L5 anterior horn cells firing and that causes extensor plantar response.

Procedure:

Stimulation of the lateral plantar aspect of the foot with the blunt end of the patellar hammer or key from the heel to the toes, and across the metatarsal pads to the base of the big toe. Avoid touching the ball of the big toe.

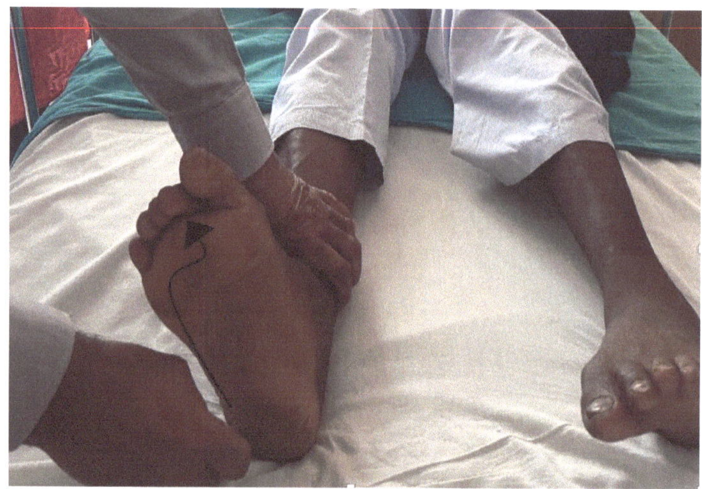

Figure B.f.1: Demonstrating plantar reflex.

Components of Babinski reflex:

- Dorsiflexion or upward movement of the big toe.
- Fanning of the other toes.
- Dorsiflexion at ankle
- Flexion at knee
- Contraction of tensor fascia lata and flexion and hip joint

Other method to elicit Babinski sign:

- Chaddock (stimulating under lateral malleolus)
- Gordon (squeezing calf)
- Oppenhiem (applying pressure to the medial side of the tibia)

The Hoffmann reflex in the upper extremity is considered the nearest equivalent to the babinski sign.

Clinical significance:

- Present in the lesion of corticospinal tract/pyramidal tract/upper motor lesion
- Infants up to 24 months of age
- When a patient is asleep

g. Abdominal reflex

Table B.g.1: Checklist

Type of Station: Eliciting the abdominalreflex in the patient
Domain: Cognitive, Psychomotor, Affective.
Communication Time: 1 minute

Marks-10

Sr. no	Steps	Marks	Roll.no
I	**Checklist**		
1.	Stands on the right side of the subject and makes subject comfortable in lying down position and explained the procedure.	1	
2.	Expose the abdomen above up to the xiphisternum and below up to pubic symphysis	1	
3.	Stroking the abdominal wall with pointed end of patellar hammer in each of the four quadrants of the abdomen.	1	
4.	Stroking diagonally towards the umbilicus in each of the four quadrants of the abdomen.	1	
5.	Looked for contractions of abdominal muscle in each quadrant	1	
6.	Looked for Beevor's sign – asked the patients to perform a quarter sit-up with the arms crossed behind the head	1	
7.	Watched the umbilicus movement.	1	
8.	Able to interpret like Beevor's sign is considered positive, if the navel moves up, down, or to either side.	1	
II	**Assessment of Professional Behavior**		
1	Addressed patient appropriately and introduced himself/herself by name	1	
2	Informed patient regarding completion of the procedure and thanked the patient before leaving	1	
III	**Total Marks (Tick)**	10	
	Final Score		
	Global Rating: 1. Poor; 2. Unsatisfactory; 3. Satisfactory; 4. Good; 5. Excellent		
	Observer's Comment (based on general observation):		
	Signature of the Observer		

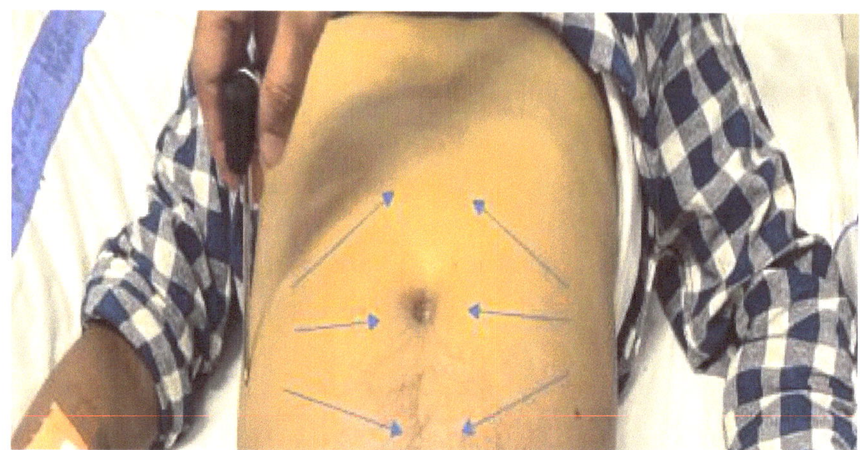

Figure B.g.1: Demonstrating abdominal reflex

Root Value: Upper abdominal reflexes are supplied by nerve roots T9-T11. Lower abdominal reflexes are supplied by roots T11-T12.

Procedure: These reflexes can be tested by lightly stroking the abdominal wall diagonally towards the umbilicus in each of the four quadrants of the abdomen.

Reflex contractions of the abdominal wall are absent in upper motor neuron lesions above the segmental level and also in patients who have had surgical operations interrupting the nerves.

They can also be absent in normal people with lax abdomen.

Beevor's sign: Patients perform a quarter sit-up with the arms crossed behind the head. The students should be watching the umbilicus movement. Beevor's sign is considered positive if the navel moves up, down, or to either side.

h. Cremastric reflex

Table B.h.1: Checklist

Type of Station: Eliciting the cremasteric reflex in the patient
Domain: Cognitive, Psychomotor, Affective.
Communication Time: 1 minute

Marks-10

Sr. no	Steps	Marks	Roll.no
I	**Checklist**		
1	Stands on the right side of the subject and makesthesubject comfortable in lying down position and explains the procedure.	1	
2	Expose the genital area completely with the thigh apart	1	
3	Stroking the medial part of the thigh in a downward direction.	1	
4	Looked for the cremasteric muscle contractions	1	
5	Looked for pulling the scrotum and testis superiorly on the side	1	
6	Whether elicited by other methods like pressing over the sartorius in the lower third of Hunter's canal.	1	
7	Root value and clinical significance	1	
8	Looked the same on the other side	1	
II	**Assessment of Professional Behavior**		
1	Addressed the patient appropriately and introduced himself/herself by name	1	
2	Informed patient regarding completion of the procedure and thanked the patient before leaving	1	
III	**Total Marks (Tick)**	10	
	Final Score		
	Global Rating: 1. Poor; 2. Unsatisfactory; 3. Satisfactory; 4. Good; 5. Excellent		
	Observer's Comment (based on general observation):		
	Signature of the Observer		

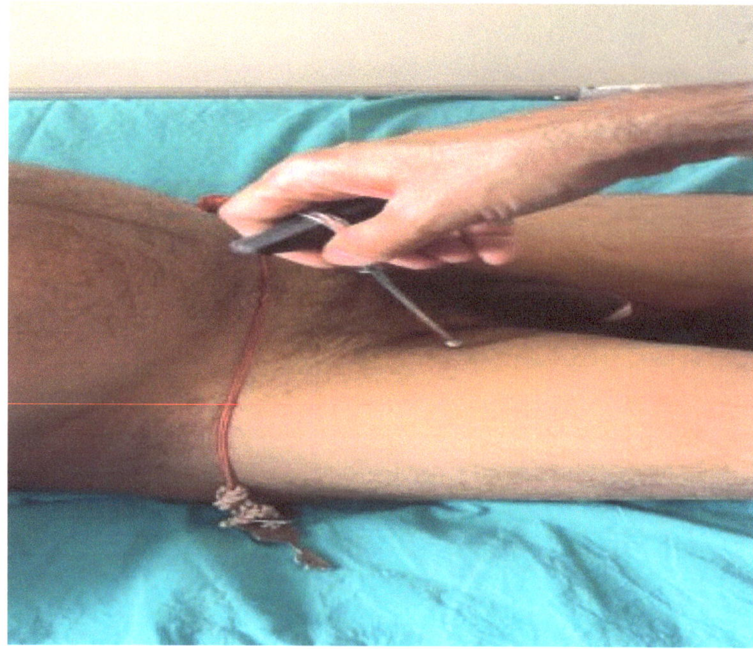

Figure B.h.1: Demonstrating cremasteric reflex

The cremasteric reflex is a superficial reflex present in males.

Root value: It evaluates the function of the cremasteric muscle which is supplied by the genitofemoral nerve (L1, L2).

Procedure: This reflex is elicited by stroking the medial part of the thigh in a downward direction. In a normal response, the cremasteric muscle contracts, thereby pulling the scrotum and testis superiorly on the side that is assessed.

The cremasteric reflex can often be more easily elicited by pressing over the sartorius in the lower third of Hunter's canal.

The female equivalent of this test is called the **Geigel reflex**. In females, there is a contraction of muscle fibers above the superior border of the inguinal ligament. Hence, it is sometimes referred to as the inguinal reflex.

C. Sensory Examination

a. Cortical sensations

Table C.a.1: Checklist
Type of Station: Procedural station
Check for cortical sensations in the patient.
Domain: Cognitive, Psychomotor, Affective.
Communication Time: 1 minute   Marks 10

Sr. no	Steps	Marks	Roll. no
I	**Checklist**		
1.	Stands on the right side of the subject and makes subject comfortable in sitting position and explained the procedure. Ask the patient to close eyes while performing the examination.	1	
2.	Stereognosis – ability to recognize and identify objects by feeling them.	1	
3.	Graphesthesia – ability to recognize symbols, letters or numbers written on skin.	1	
4.	Two point discrimination – ability to recognize simultaneous stimulation by two sharp points.	1	
5.	Tactile localization (topognosis) – ability to localize stimuli to parts of body.	2	
6.	Examine both side	2	
II	**Assessment of Professional Behavior**		
1	Addressed the patient appropriately and introduced himself/herself by name	1	
2	Informed patient regarding completion of the procedure and thanked the patient before leaving	1	
III	**Total Marks (Tick)**	10	
	Final Score		
	Global Rating: 1. Poor; 2. Unsatisfactory; 3. Satisfactory; 4. Good; 5. Excellent		
	Observer's Comment (based on general observation)		
	Signature of the Observer		

Notes:

Clinical application

- Eliciting the presence of cortical sensations
- Knowledge of the site of the lesion
- Absence of cortical sensation causes.

Cortical sensations:

Accurate localization of stimuli and assessment of shape, weight, size, and texture of objects mediated by parietal lobes. Sensory modalities must be intact to measure cortical sensations.

Stereognosis: The ability to recognize and identify objects by feeling them. The absence of this ability is called astereognosis. Test object must be familiar, easily identifiable, and large enough for a weak hand to feel. The patient with eyes closed, is asked to identify an object placed in his hands. If he fails or takes too long to decide, it is placed on the other hand for comparison.

Graphesthesia: The ability to recognize symbols, letters, or numbers written on skin. The absence of this ability is termed graphanesthesia. The patient closes his eyes and letters or numbers are traced out on the palm, anterior forearm, thigh, or lower leg, clear finger like 8,4,5 should be used. More difficult like 3,6,9 is used as finer tests.

Two-point discrimination: Ability to recognize simultaneous stimulation by two sharp points. Measured by the distance between the points required for recognition. Finger pulp and lips – 3-5 mm separation well recognized.

Palm – 2-3 cm
Sole – 4 cm
Dorsum of foot – 5 cm and above
Legs – 5 cm and above
Back – 5 cm and above.
If two-point discrimination is lost in the presence of intact posterior column sensations, it indicates a parietal lobe lesion.

Tactile localization (topognosis): The ability to localize stimuli to parts of the body. Topagnosia is the absence of this ability. Pin or fingertip is used and the patient's eyes are closed and asked to indicate the point touched with his fingers. Painful stimuli should not be used.

Sensory extinction: The ability to perceive a sensory stimulus when corresponding areas on the opposite side of the body are stimulated simultaneously. Loss of ability is termed sensory extinction. The site of the lesion is the contralateral parietal lobe.

b. Spinothalamic tract (Pain, Touch, Temprature)

Pain:

Table C.b.1: Checklist

Type of Station: Procedural station

Eliciting the spinothalamic tract (pain) features in the patient

Domain: Cognitive, psychomotor, Affective.

Communication Time: 1 minute   Marks-10

Sr. no.	Steps	Marks	Roll.no
I	**Checklist**		
1.	Stands on the right side of the subject and makes subject comfortable in lying down position and explained the procedure.	1	
2.	Choose sharp pin with round head for testing pain	1	
3.	Choose part of patient body from history expected to be normal	1	
4.	Touch him precisely but not too firmly several times with point of the pin	1	
5.	Ask him a) if he can feel anything b) what it is that he can feel c) if he says that he can feel a point ask if it is sharp or blunt	1	
6.	Having established patient recognizes stimulus, compare appreciation of sensation in number of areas including face, shoulders, inner and outer aspects of lower forearm, thumb and little finger, upper and lower chest and abdomen, front of the thighs, lateral and medial aspect of lower legs, dorsum of feet, little toe and buttock on both sides	1	
7.	From history, attention drawn to areas likely to be abnormal and areas revealed abnormality in preliminary screening	1	
8.	Compared in both sides	1	
II	**Assessment of Professional Behavior**		
1	Addressed patient appropriately and introduced himself/herself by name	1	
2	Informed patient regarding completion of the procedure and thanked the patient before leaving	1	
III	**Total Marks (Tick)**	**10**	
	Final Score		
	Global Rating: 1. Poor; 2. Unsatisfactory; 3. Satisfactory; 4. Good; 5. Excellent		
	Observer's Comment (based on general observation):		
	Signature of the Observer		

Introduction:

Students will be evaluated for examination of signs of the spinothalamic tract. The student needs to understand the clinical technique and interpretation of signs of the spinothalamic tract.

Expected from a student:

- The student should be well apprised of the use of pins, cotton wool, tuning fork, and test tubes having hot and cold water.
- The student should be acquainted with the proper steps of the eliciting sensation.
- The student needs to be aware of the expected result and its interpretation.

Clinical Application:

- Eliciting pain sensation
- Knowledge of various other sensations

Touch

Table C.b.2: Checklist

Type of Station: Procedural station

Eliciting the spinothalamic tract (touch) features in the patient

Domain: Cognitive, psychomotor, Affective.

Communication Time: 1 minute   Marks-10

Sr. no.	Steps	Marks	Roll.no
I	**Checklist**		
1.	Stands on the right side of the subject and makes subject comfortable in lying down position and explained the procedure.	1	
2.	Choose small piece of cotton wool for testing touch	1	
3.	Choose part of patient body from history expected to be normal	1	
4.	Tell patient to shut his eyes and say 'Yes' each time he feels anything	1	
5.	Cotton wool is shaped to a point and skin is touched lightly, testing again in dermatome areas	1	
6.	Having established patient recognizes stimulus, compare appreciation of sensation in number of areas including face, shoulders, inner and outer aspects of lower forearm, thumb and little finger, upper and lower chest and abdomen, front of the thighs, lateral and medial aspect of lower legs, dorsum of feet, little toe and buttock on both sides	1	
7.	From history, attention drawn to areas likely to be abnormal and areas revealed abnormality in preliminary screening	1	
8.	Mark the point and change the direction of cotton wool, always move from impaired to normal sensation.	1	
II	**Assessment of Professional Behavior**		
1	Addressed patient appropriately and introduced himself/herself by name	1	
2	Informed patient regarding completion of the procedure and thanked the patient before leaving	1	
III	**Total Marks (Tick)**	10	
	Final Score		
	Global Rating: 1. Poor; 2. Unsatisfactory; 3. Satisfactory; 4. Good; 5. Excellent		
	Observer's Comment (based on general observation):		
	Signature of the Observer		

Clinical application:

- Eliciting touch sensation
- Knowledge of various other sensations

Temperature:

Table C.b.3: Checklist

Type of Station: Procedural station

Eliciting the spinothalamic tract (temperature) features in the patient

Domain: Cognitive, psychomotor, Affective.

Communication Time: 1 minute   Marks-10

Sr. no.	Steps	Marks	Roll.no
I	**Checklist**		
1.	Stands on the right side of the subject and makes subject comfortable in lying down position and explained the procedure.	1	
2.	For preliminary screening, patient can compare temperature of a cold object such as tuning fork on main sensory area of body	1	
3.	After this, use test tubes containing hot water and cold water	1	
4.	Tell patient to shut his eyes and ask what he can feel	1	
5.	Whether there is any difference when other tube is used and what the difference is.	1	
6.	Having established patient recognizes stimulus, compare appreciation of sensation in number of areas including face, shoulders, inner and outer aspects of lower forearm, thumb and little finger, upper and lower chest and abdomen, front of the thighs, lateral and medial aspect of lower legs, dorsum of feet, little toe and buttock on both sides	1	
7.	From history, attention drawn to areas likely to be abnormal and areas revealed abnormality in preliminary screening	1	
8.	Always move from impaired to normal sensation and compared on both sides also	1	
II	**Assessment of Professional Behavior**		
1	Addressed patient appropriately and introduced himself/herself by name	1	
2	Informed patient regarding completion of the procedure and thanked the patient before leaving	1	
III	**Total Marks (Tick)**	**10**	
	Final Score		
	Global Rating: 1. Poor; 2. Unsatisfactory; 3. Satisfactory; 4. Good; 5. Excellent		
	Observer's Comment (based on general observation):		

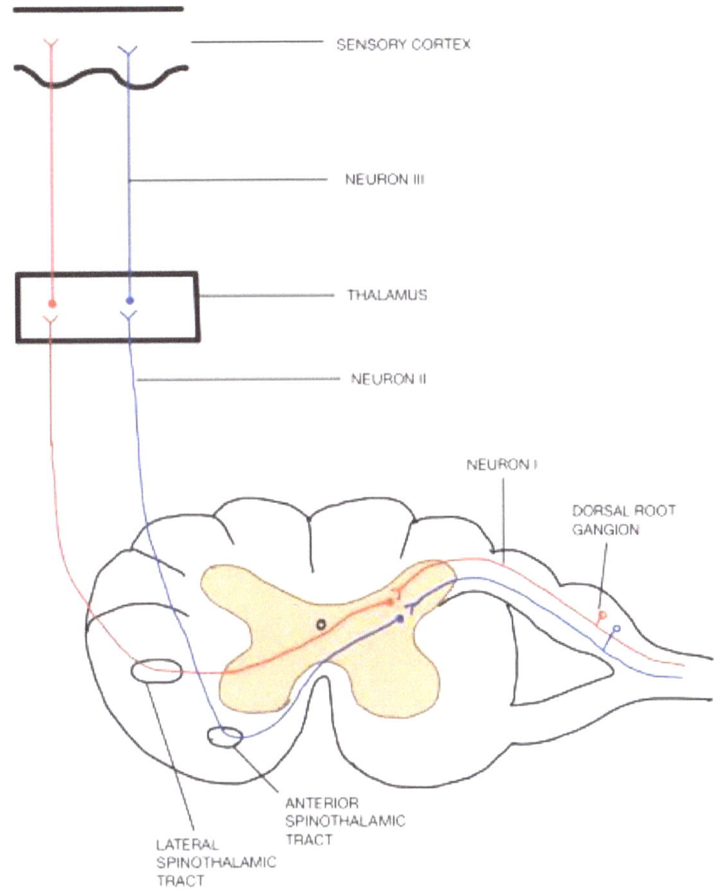

Figure C.b.1: Showing the Lateral and Anterior Spinothalamic tract pathway

Note:

The lateralspinothalamic tract carries pain and temperature sensations from the whole and opposite half of the body except the head and neck where sensations are carried by V, IX, and X cranial nerves.

Patterns of Sensory loss:

Total unilateral loss of all forms of sensation including face: Thalamus

Ipsilateral loss of facial sensation with contralateral loss of pain and temperature sensation over body: lateral medullary syndrome

Loss of all modalities of sensation below a level over trunk: transverse myelopathy

Loss of pain and temperature sensation below a level on the contralateral side and loss of position and vibration sense below the level on the ipsilateral side: Brown Sequard Syndrome

Loss of sensation of 'saddle' type: Cauda conus syndrome

Glove and stocking anaesthesia: peripheral polyneuropathy

Loss of all forms of sensation over a clearly defined area in one part of the body only: radiculopathy, mononeuritis multiplex, mononeuropathy

c. Posterior Column Examination (Vibration Sense, Position Sense)

Table C.c.1: Checklist

Type of Station: Procedural station
Eliciting the Posterior Column (Vibration Sense, Position Sense)
Domain: Cognitive, Psychomotor, Affective.
Communication Time: 1 minute   Marks-10

Sr. no.	Steps	Marks	Roll.no
I	**Checklist**		
1.	Stands on the right side of the subject and makes subject comfortable in lying down position and explained the procedure.	1	
2.	Put the vibrating tuning fork (128 Hz) on the bony prominences like dorsum of the big toe and medial malleolus then tibial tuberosity.	1	
3.	Compared on the other lower limb as well.	1	
4.	Put the vibrating tuning fork (128 Hz) on the vertebral spine	1	
5.	Hold the proximal phalanx with one thumb and finger and hold the medial and lateral sides of the distal phalanx with the fingers of the other hand. Move the distal phalanx up and down and ask the patient with eyes opened and to identify the movement.	1	
6.	Hold the proximal phalanx with one thumb and finger and hold the medial and lateral sides of the distal phalanx with the fingers of the other hand. Move the distal phalanx up and down and ask the patient to close his eyes and to identify the movement.	1	
7.	Also replicate this movement in every joint	1	
8.	Looked for Romberg's Sign by asking the patient to stand with eyes closed and both hands apart	1	
II	**Assessment of Professional Behavior**		
1	Addressed patient appropriately and introduced himself/herself by name	1	
2	Informed patient regarding completion of the procedure and thanked the patient before leaving	1	
III	**Total Marks (Tick)**	**10**	
	Final Score		
	Global Rating: 1. Poor; 2. Unsatisfactory; 3. Satisfactory; 4. Good; 5. Excellent		
	Observer's Comment (based on general observation):		

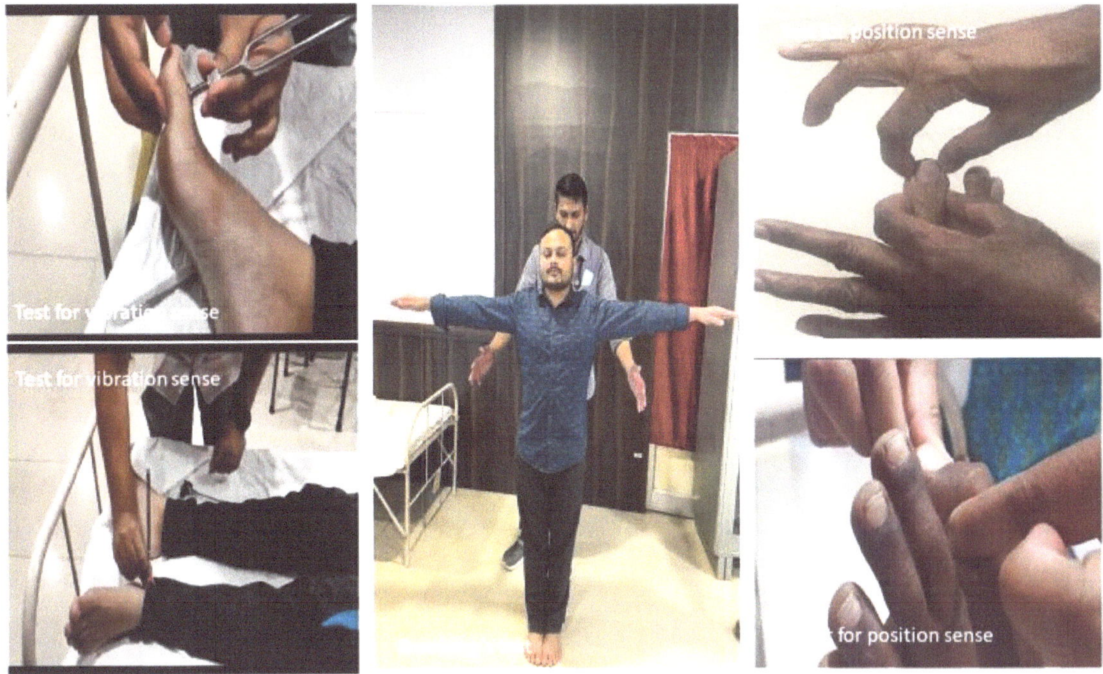

Figure C.c.1: Demonstrating Posterior Column Examination

Introduction

- Posterior column consists of fasciculus gracilis and fasciculus cuneatus.
- Entry of axons is from posterior root ganglion and exits through posterior white column of same side which further bifurcates into long ascending and short descending branches.
- Ascending fibres are fasciculus gracilis and fasciculus cuneatus.
- Fasciculus gracilis contains fibers from the sacral, lumbar, and lower six thoracic spinal nerves. Fasciculus cuneatus contains fibers from the upper six thoracic and all cervical spinal nerves.
- Impression of vibration sense and position of different parts of the body can be recognized.
- Many second-orderneurons of fasciculus cuneatus enter the cerebellum through the inferior cerebellar peduncle of the same side. This is the cuneo-cerebellar tract and fibers are called posterior external arcuatefibers.
- Muscle joint sense is conveyed through these fibers to the cerebellum.

Clinical application

- Eliciting defect of the posterior column.
- Knowledge of the site of the lesion
- Knowledge of loss of proprioception.
- Different pathways

Notes

Position sense and sense of passive movement are two closely related sensations. Where most people refer to the test of position sense or joint sense.

Position sense

Procedure:ask the patient to close their eye throughout the procedure. Place the patient's arm in a particular position, then move it away and ask him first to replace it himself, and then to place the opposite limb in a similar position. Ask him to touch the forefinger of one hand with the forefinger of the other, and make it harder by moving his finger to different positions. Let him try adopting similar positions with his legs, and ask him to touch his outstretched hand with his big toe. Ask him to place his forefinger accurately on the tip of his nose, and his heel accurately on his knee.

Sense of passive movement

Procedure: The patient's eye must be closed. The digit [thumb, finger, or big toe] is held firmly and moved up and down, while the patient is asked if he can feel the movement. If so, he should be told that he is going to be asked whether his thumb has been moved upwards or downwards. Move the digit widely in the appropriate directions so that he understands which movement he is calling 'up' and which 'down'.

Hold sides of digits between finger and thumb, so that uneven pressure above or below does not reveal the direction of movement, and make a clear and precise movement in one or other direction.

Repeat the test several times avoiding alternate movements, and if any error is made, the test should be continued until at least six successive correct responses are given or until one is satisfied that the defect is constant.

If digit movement cannot be detected in the first place, the same test is carried out at the wrist, elbow, and knee.

If one suspectsavery minor defect, the test can be varied by asking the patient to say 'now' at the movement he feels the toe moving. The defect can be so gross that the patient has no knowledge of wide displacement at the shoulder or hip.

Vibration

Procedure:

A tuning fork (128 Hz) of well-maintained vibration is shown to the patient and then placed on his clavicle to allow him to identify the sensation of the vibration.

He then closes his eyes, the fork is struck and placed on bony points starting from the internal malleolus and lower end of the radius. If there is gross deficiency here then it can be placed on tibial tuberosity and elbow, ASIS, and clavicle.

the patient is first asked if he can feel the vibrations the fork is stopped by touching it and the speed with which he recognized is noted. Two sides are now compared first by asking whether the degree of vibration feels the same and then by comparing the promptness with which he notes the sensation of vibration.

d. Cerebellar Examination

Table C.d.1: Checklist

Type of Station: Procedural station
Eliciting the Cerebellar Signs
Domain: Cognitive, Psychomotor, Affective.
Communication Time: 1 minute   Marks-10

Sr. no.	Steps	Marks	Roll.no
I	**Checklist**		
1.	Stands in front of the subject and makes subject comfortable in sitting position and explained the procedure.	1	
2.	Elicit the rebound phenomenon by flexing the subject's arm at elbow against resistance and examiner placing his other hand in front of patient's face to avoid injury.	1	
3.	Elicit finger nose finger test by asking patient alternatively touch his index finger to his nose and examiner's finger.	1	
4.	Examined for dysdiadochokinesia by alternating pronation and supination of the hand, by striking on the other palm.	1	
5.	Eliciting pendular jerk by striking on the patellar tendon, with patient in sitting position and feet hanging freely. And seeing the pendular movements more than 3 times.	1	
6.	Looked for the tandem walking by asking the patient to walk on straight line by keeping the heel of one foot in front of the toe of other foot and look for swaying.	1	
7.	Looked for Heel to Shin test by asking patient to flex hip of one limb and slide heel smoothly down the crest of tibial shin to ankle of the other lower limb.	1	
8.	Looked for titubation in the trunk by asking the patient to sit on the bed.	1	
II	**Assessment of Professional Behavior**		
1	Addressed patient appropriately and introduced himself/herself by name	1	
2	Informed patient regarding completion of the procedure and thanked the patient before leaving	1	
III	**Total Marks (Tick)**	**10**	
	Final Score		
	Global Rating: 1. Poor; 2. Unsatisfactory; 3. Satisfactory; 4. Good; 5. Excellent		
	Observer's Comment (based on general observation):		

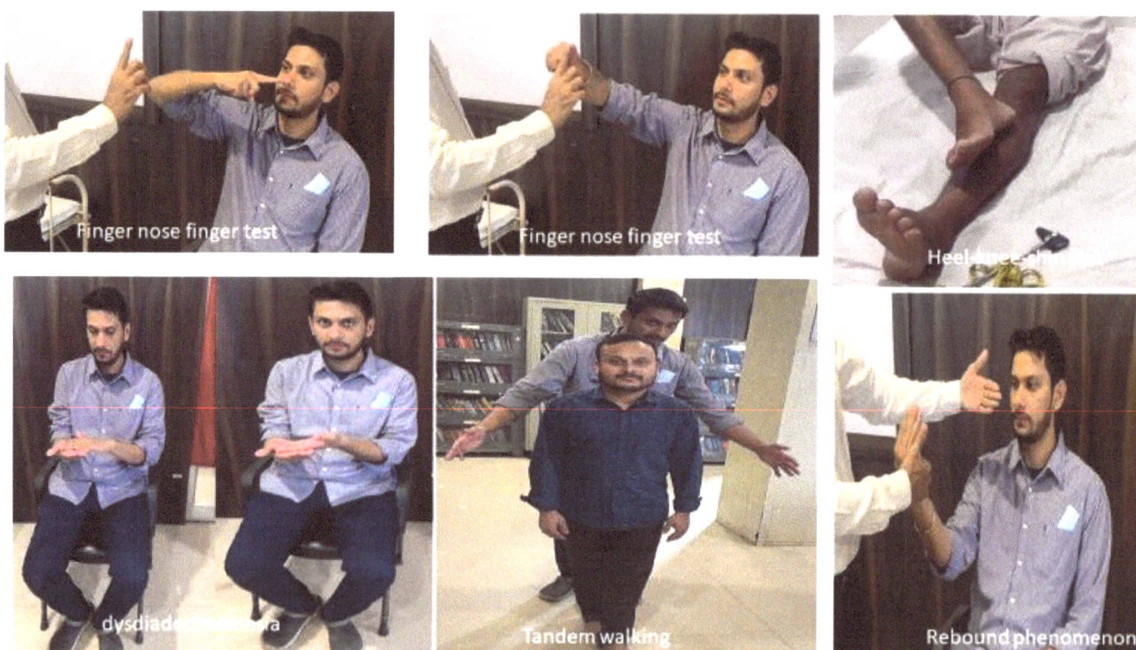

Figure C.d.1: Demonstrating Cerebellar Signs

Introduction-

Hypotonia: Ipsilateral to the side of a cerebellar lesion. More noticeable in the upper limbs and proximal muscles.

Pendular knee jerk: Leg keeps swinging after knee jerk more than 3 times (3 or less is considered normal).

Dysmetria: Finger-to-nose test – With eyes open, the patient is asked to partially extend their elbow and rapidly bring the tip of their index finger in a wide arc to the tip of his nose.

Heel-to-shin test – The patient is asked to place one heel on the opposite knee and slide the heel down the tibia with the foot dorsiflexed. Movement should be performed accurately. In cerebellar disease, the arc of the movement is jerky/wavering.

Dysdiadochokinesia: Alternating movements (pronate and supinate forearm and hand quickly): In cerebellar disease, the movements tend to overshoot or are inadequate resulting in irregular or inaccurate movements.

Stewart-Holmes rebound sign – Have the patient pull on your hand and when they do, slip your hand out of their grasp. A positive sign is seen in cerebellar disease, be careful that you protect the patient from the unrestricted movement causing them to strike themselves.

Cerebellar dysarthria: Scanning speech, in which there is the enunciation of individual syllables: "the British Parliament" becomes "the Brit-trish Par-la-ment." Local twisting language may be tired like MATA CHA SATARA, which becomes MA-TA-CHA – SA – TA-RA.

Intention tremor: Occurs during goal-directed movements. Intention tremor results when the antagonist activation that normally stops a goal-directed movement as the goal is approached is inappropriately sized or timed.

Oculomotor dysfunction: Nystagmusis frequently seen in cerebellar disorders. Gaze-evoked nystagmus, upbeat nystagmus, rebound nystagmus, and optokineticnystagmus may all be seen in midline cerebellar lesions.

Gait: The gait is ataxic if the patient sways towards the side of the lesion. In the vermis lesion, there is truncal ataxia. Titubation Consists of a rhythmic body or head tremor. There is a rotatory, rocking, or bobbing movement. Clinically, this does not have significant value in localizing the lesion concerning the part of the cerebellum involved.

D. Demonstration of Meningeal Signs

Table D.1: Checklist

Type of Station: Procedural station
Eliciting the examination of Meningeal signs
Domain: Cognitive, Psychomotor, Affective.
Communication Time: 1 minute   Marks-10

Sr. no	Steps	Marks	R.no
I	**Checklist**		
1	Stands on the right side of the subject and makesthesubject comfortable in lying down position and explains the procedure.	1	
2	To flex the neck so that the chin of the face touches the chest and feels for the resistance of the movement	1	
3	Feels the resistance while extending the knee in a flexed hip (Kernig's sign)	2	
4	While flexing the neck, note the flexion in the hip and knee (Brudzenski's neck sign)	2	
5	While flexing the leg at the knee joint, there will be flexion at the knee joint in the other limb (Brudzenski's leg sign)	2	
II	**Assessment of Professional Behavior**		
1	Addressed the patient appropriately and introduced himself/herself by name	1	
2	Informed patient regarding completion of the procedure and thanked the patient before leaving	1	
III	**Total Marks (Tick)**	10	
	Final Score		
	Global Rating: 1. Poor; 2. Unsatisfactory; 3. Satisfactory; 4. Good; 5. Excellent		
	Observer's Comment (based on general observation):		
	Signature of the Observer		

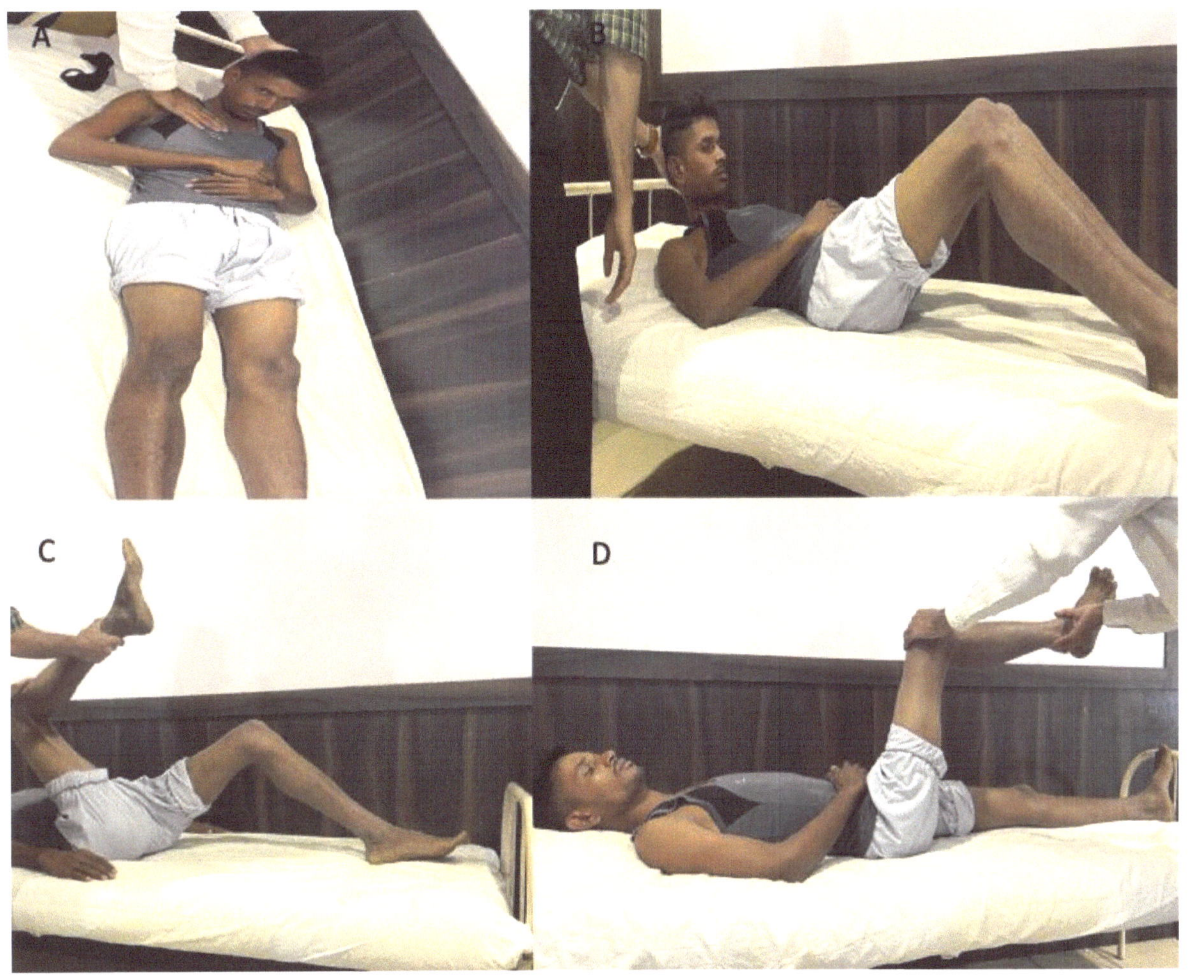

Figure D.1 –
A: Demonstrating testing for neck rigidity/stiffness
B: Demonstrating Brudzinski'sneck sign
C: Demonstrating Brudzinski'sleg sign
D: ShowingKernig's Sign

Introduction:

Students will be evaluated for demonstration of Meningeal signs. The student needs to understand the clinical technique and interpretation of Kernig's and Brudzenski's signs. Meningeal signs are elicited most frequently when the meninges are inflamed.

Expected from a student:

- The student should be acquainted with the proper steps of eliciting the meningeal signs.
- The student needs to be aware of the expected result and its interpretation.

Clinical application:

- Eliciting the Meningeal signs
- Knowledge of Meningismus

Notes:

Meningeal signs:

Meningeal signs are elicited in general when the meninges are inflamed either from infection (Bacterial Meningitis) or from foreign material (Blood in subarachnoid space). Meningismus is the term that refers to the presence of neck rigidity and other meningeal signs. Meningism is the term given to the presence of neck rigidity/stiffness in the absence of meningeal inflammation. It is usually seen in younger children with systemic infections. The general clinical manifestations of inflamed meninges include neck stiffness, irritability, photophobia, nausea, and vomiting along with the presence or absence of fever and chills.

Neck stiffness:

It is the most commonly encountered sign of meningitis. It is characterized by stiffness and spasms of neck muscles. There can sometimes be resistance to passive flexion or marked spasms of muscles. The physician cannot place the patient's chin on his chest, but there is no marked difficulty in hyperextending the neck.

Other causes of Neck Rigidity:

- Cervical spondylosis
- Retropharyngeal abscess
- Neck trauma
- Cervical Lymphadenopathy

Kernig's sign:

The common method of eliciting this sign is to flex the hip and then knee to right angles and then to passively extend the knee which produces pain, resistance, and inability to completely extend the knee.

Brudzinski's sign:

Placing the hand under the patient's head in an attempt to flex the neck causes flexion of the knees and hips bilaterally. The Brudzinski's leg sign or contralateral leg sign is elicited by flexing one hip and knee and the contralateral leg undergoes flexion.

E. Demonstration of Straight Leg Raising Test

Table E.1: Checklist

Type of Station: Procedural station
Eliciting the examination of the Straight Leg Rising test
Domain: Cognitive, Psychomotor, Affective.
Communication Time: 1 minute   Marks-10

Sr. no	Steps	Marks	R.no
I	**Checklist**		
1	Stands on the right side of the subject and makesthesubject comfortable in lying down position and explains the procedure.	1	
2	Look for the Lasegue sign	2	
3	Raise the extended leg and feel for the limitation in doing so towards the side of the lesion	2	
4	Observe the patient's face for pain	2	
5	Repeats the procedure in the other leg	1	
II	**Assessment of Professional Behavior**		
1	Addressed the patient appropriately and introduced himself/herself by name	1	
2	Informed patient regarding completion of the procedure and thanked the patient before leaving	1	
III	**Total Marks (Tick)**	10	
	Final Score		
	Global Rating: 1. Poor; 2. Unsatisfactory; 3. Satisfactory; 4. Good; 5. Excellent		
	Observer's Comment (based on general observation):		
	Signature of the Observer		

Introduction:

Students will be evaluated for demonstration of the Straight leg raising test. The student needs to understand the clinical technique of the Straight leg raising test. The student should understand the difference betweenthe Straight leg raising test and Kernig's sign.

Expected from a student:

- The student should be acquainted with the proper steps of eliciting the straight-legraising test.
- The student needs to be aware of the expected result and its interpretation.

Clinical application:

- Know the causes of Radiculopathy
- Assessment and interpretation of the straight-legraising test

Procedure:

This is a test that is done to elicit the presence of L4, L5, or S1 Radiculopathy

This test is done with the patient lying in the supine position and the heel of the leg is elevated slowly the test is considered positive if sciatic pain is reproduced between 35 degrees to 70 degrees

Lasegue sign is a test for lower lumbosacral root irritation for conditions like disc prolapse. Lasegue sign is sometimes used synonymously with the Straight leg raising test.

The **Reverse SLR** test is a way of eliciting root stretch in the evaluation of high lumbar radiculopathy. The patient is made to lie in the prone position and the knee is pulled into maximum flexion.

There is some overlap between Kernig's sign and the Straight leg raising sign. The technique has slight similarity. The technique is similar but the Straight leg raising test is used to check for root irritation in Lumbosacral radiculopathy. In cases of Meningitis, both Kernig's sign and straight leg rising sign are positive. But in cases of Radiculopathy of one side, the Straight leg raising sign is positive on only one side. A bilateral positive straight leg raising test should raise suspicion of meningitis.

Chapter 3

Respiratory System

A. Palpation of Trachea

Table A.1: Checklist

Type of Station: Procedural station
Palpating the Trachea in the patient
Domain: Cognitive, Psychomotor, Affective.
Communication Time: 1 minute

Marks-10

Sr. no	Steps	Marks	Roll.no
I	**Checklist**		
1	Stands infront of the subject and makes the subject comfortable, and explains the procedure	1	
2	Exposes the neck of the patient	1	
3	Flexes the Head of the patient slightly	1	
4	Placed the index finger and ring finger over the two sternoclavicularjoints.	1	
5	Palpated the thyroid cartilage using the middle finger	1	
6	Traced the trachea downwards from the thyroid cartilage	1	
7	Looked for the crico-sternal distance	1	
8	Practiced the insinuation method	1	
II	**Assessment of Professional Behavior**		
1	Addressed the patient appropriately and introduced himself/herself by name	1	
2	Informed patient regarding completion of the procedure and thanked the patient before leaving	1	
III	**Total Marks (Tick)**	**10**	
	Final Score		
	Global Rating: 1. Poor; 2. Unsatisfactory; 3. Satisfactory; 4. Good; 5. Excellent		
	Observer's Comment (based on general observation):		
	Signature of the Observer		

Introduction:

The ability to palpate the trachea will be used to evaluate students. The learner must comprehend the clinical procedure and interpretation for tracheal palpation.

- The larynx and the bronchi of the lungs are connected by the cartilaginous tube known as the trachea.
- The trachea eventually divides into the left and right major bronchus at the carina, which is where it starts at the bottom margin of the cricoid cartilage of the larynx.
- The trachea starts at the level of C6, and the carina is located at C4; however, during the process of respiration, the position of the carina may change.
- The patient might be seated or standing while being asked to tilt their chin downward to relax the neck muscles in preparation for tracheal palpation.
- The examiner's middle finger is used to trace the trachea from the cricoid cartilage downward while the index and ring fingers are placed on the sternoclavicular joints.
- The examiner should use their fingers to measure the distance between the suprasternal notch to the cricoid cartilage to determine the cricosternal distance. To find the area lateral to the trachea, which needs to be compared on both sides, the examiner inserts the middle finger into the space between the trachea and the medial border of the sternocleidomastoid muscle using the insinuation technique.
- In healthy individuals, three fingers can be readily placed in this space, but in emphysema patients, the mediastinum is dragged down and the lung is hyperinflated; as a result, the crico-sternal distance is lowered and is less than three fingers.

Expected from a student:

- The student should be well-versed in the method of tracheal palpation and should help the patient attain the proper position by flexing the head
- The student should be acquainted with the proper steps of palpating the trachea
- The student needs to be aware of the expected results and the interpretation of the result

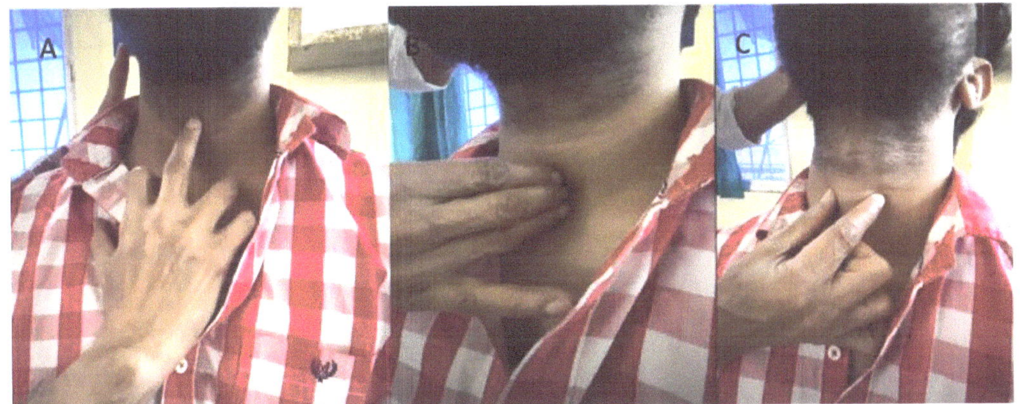

Figure A.1 – A: Demonstrating the method of palpation of the trachea
B: Demonstrating insinuation method
C: Testing for Tracheal Tug

Clinical Application:

- Palpating the trachea
- Assessing if the trachea is central or deviated

A difference in the amount of space on the two sides of the trachea suggests deviation of the trachea.

- Palpating the crico-sternal distance
- Knowing the causes of tracheal deviation and abnormal crico-sternal distance

Notes:

The trachea is deviated to the side of pathology in cases of:

Lung Collapse
Pneumonectomy
Unilateral Fibrosis of the Lung
Agenesis of the lung (Complete absence of the whole lung along with its bronchus)

The trachea is deviated to the opposite side of pathology in cases of:

Tension Pneumothorax
Pleural Effusion
Mediastinal Mass
Para-tracheal mass

Campbell's Sign:

One finger is placed over the cricoid cartilage and this finger is noticed to move downwards during each inspiration which can be seen in cases of acute exacerbation of chronic obstructive pulmonary disease.

Oliver Sign:

A tracheal tug or Oliver sign is characteristic of the presence of an aneurysm of the arch of the aorta due to the location of the arch of the aorta over the left main bronchus. The patient's neck is hyperextended, and the cricoid cartilage is palpated, held, and pushed forward. An upward thrust is provided and now the examiner can feel systolic pulsation from the aneurysm of the arch of the aorta. An alternative method is when the patient's head is resting over the examiner's chest and both the index fingers from either side are used to hold the cricoid cartilage and look for systolic pulsations.

B. Tactile Vocal Fremitus

Table B.1: Checklist

Type of Station: Procedural station
Eliciting the examination of Tactile Vocal Fremitus
Domain: Cognitive, Psychomotor, Affective
Communication Time: 1 minute   Marks-10

Sr. no	Steps	Marks	R.no
I	**Checklist**		
1	Stands in front of the subject and makes the subject comfortable in a sitting position and explains the procedure.	1	
2	Exposed the chest wall fully up to the umbilicus for better examination	1	
3	Ask the patient to repeat "Ninety-Nine" or "One, two, three" in the same tone.	1	
4	Uses the ulnar border to assess the vibrations felt on the chest wall in intercostal spaces	2	
5	Repeats the procedure on the other side of the chest and covers all major portions of the chest every time	2	
6	Correctly interpreted and narrated findings to the examiner	1	
II	**Assessment of Professional Behavior**		
1	Addressed the patient appropriately and introduced himself/herself by name	1	
2	Informed patient regarding completion of the procedure and thanked the patient before leaving	1	
III	**Total Marks (Tick)**	10	
	Final Score		
	Global Rating: 1. Poor; 2. Unsatisfactory; 3. Satisfactory; 4. Good; 5. Excellent		
	Observer's Comment (based on general observation):		
	Signature of the Observer		

Introduction:

Students will be graded on their ability to demonstrate tactile vocal fremitus, which entails palpating various parts of the chest wall as the patient repeatedly repeats a word or number (such as "ninety-nine"). The learner must comprehend the clinical procedure and how to interpret test results for the tactile vocal fremitus. The strength with which the patient's voice is transferred as vibrations through the chest wall to the examiner's hands is impacted by the presence of increased tissue density or fluid.

Expected from a student:

- The student should be acquainted with the proper steps of eliciting the examination of tactile vocal fremitus.
- The student needs to be aware of the expected result and its interpretation and enlist causes of more pronounced and decreased tactile vocal fremitus

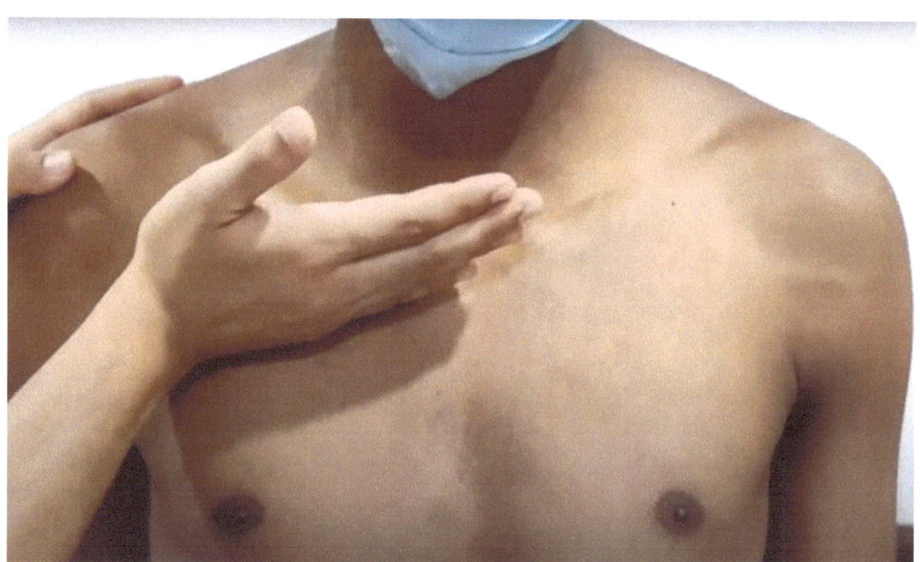

Figure B.1: Demonstrating the method to look for tactile vocal fremitus

Clinical application:

Voice fremitus is the term for the vibrations produced by the vocal cords in the tracheobronchial tree and carried to the lungs and chest wall where they can be felt (tactile fremitus).

Abnormal Tactile Vocal Fremitus

- Increased tissue density is indicated by increased vibration across that area (e.g. consolidation, tumor, lobar collapse).
- A decreased vibration across a region could be an indication of fluid or air outside the lung (e.g. pleural effusion, pneumothorax).

C. Upper Border of Liver Dullness

Table C.1: Checklist

Type of Station: Procedural station
The upper border of liver dullness and cardiac dullness
Domain: Cognitive, Psychomotor, Affective.
Communication Time: 1 minute   Marks-10

Sr. no	Steps	Marks	R.no
I	**Checklist**		
1	Stood on the Right side of the patient,makes the subject comfortable in lying down position.and Explained the procedure to the patient	1	
2	Ensure that his own hands are warm and ask the subject to breathe quietly.	1	
3	Exposed the abdomen as well as chest	1	
4	Detection of the upper border of the liver by percussing on the right side of the chest from the 6th intercostal space	2	
5	Asked the patient to take deep inspiration	2	
6	Addressed the findings	1	
B	**Assessment of Professional Behavior**		
1.	Addressed the patient appropriately and introduced himself/herself by name.	1	
2.	Informed patient regarding completion of the procedure and thanked the patient before leaving	1	
III	**Total Marks (Tick)**	10	
	Final Score		
	Global Rating: 1. Poor; 2. Unsatisfactory; 3. Satisfactory; 4. Good; 5. Excellent		
	Observer's Comment (based on general observation):		
	Signature of the Observer		

Introduction:

Students will be graded on their ability to mark the upper border of liver dullness and comprehend its clinical significance. The student must be able to interpret the upper border of liver dullness using a clinical approach.

The upper border of a healthy liver is located at the fifth intercostal gap, where the note is dull. The bottom boundary is located at or just below the right subcostal margin, and it reaches down there. The usual drabness is lessened in:

- Severe emphysema
- Large right pneumothorax
- Gas or air in the peritoneal cavity (perforation of a viscus)

Liver span: From the fifth rib, or below the right nipple in men, to the palpable right border or costal margin, the liver measures 12–15 cm in height. To determine shrinkage or expansion, serial measurements are taken.

Expected from a student:

1. The student should be aware of the steps of marking the upper border of liver dullness
2. The student should be aware of the method for the same.
3. The student should be able to correlate any abnormal findings with other clinical symptoms and signs.
4. The student should be acquainted with the proper steps of the measurement of liver span.

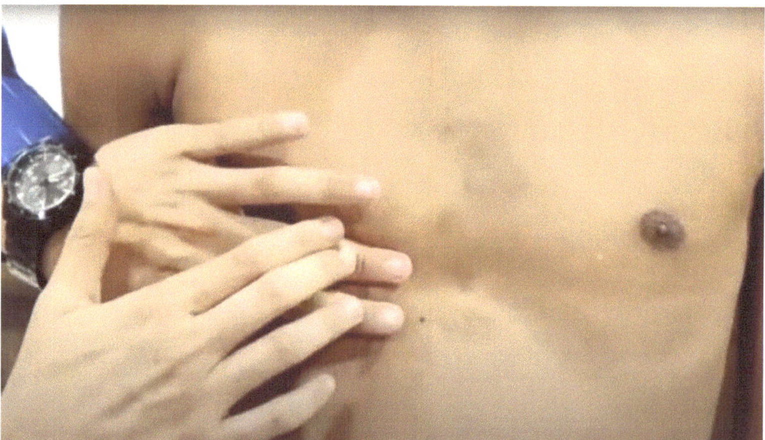

Figure C.1: Demonstrating the method to percuss the upper border of liver dullness

You should percussion the anterior chest wall along the right MCL from above downwards to define the upper border of liver dullness. In the right 5th ICS at MCL, the top border of liver dullness is typically evident.

Lowered or obliterated liver dullness is noted in:

- Emphysema.
- Pneumothorax (right-sided).
- Perforation of abdominal hollow viscus e.g. perforation of peptic ulcer.
- Cirrhosis of the liver (liver becomes small).

Elevated liver dullness:

- Amoebic or pyogenic liver abscess.
- Sub diaphragmatic abscess (right).
- Pleural effusion (right).
- Basal pneumonia (right).
- Increased intraabdominal tension due to ascites or pregnancy.

The upper border of liver dullness is present in the right 7th and 9th ICS when percussed along midaxillary and scapular line respectively.

D. Traube's Space Percussion

Table D.1: Checklist

Type of Station: Procedural station
Examination of Traube's space
Domain: Cognitive, Psychomotor, Affective.
Communication Time: 1 minute

Marks-10

Sr No	Steps	Marks	R.no
I	**Checklist**		
1	Stands on the right side of the subject and makes the subject comfortable in lying down position and explains the procedure.	1	
2	Expose the patient from the thorax to the umbilicus	1	
3	Identified the 2nd Intercostal space by palpation.	1	
4	After identifying the 2nd intercostal space, counted till the 6th rib with an imaginary line perpendicular to the subcostal arch	2	
5	In the anterior axillary line,thepatient percussed from the 9th rib to the subcostal arch	2	
6	Marked the rectangular space and summarize the Percussion finding of the rectangular space	1	
II	**Assessment of Professional Behavior**		
1	Addressed the patient appropriately and introduced himself/herself by name	1	
2	Informed patient regarding completion of the procedure and thanked the patient before leaving	1	
III	**Total Marks (Tick)**	10	
	Final Score		
	Global Rating: 1. Poor; 2. Unsatisfactory; 3. Satisfactory; 4. Good; 5. Excellent		
	Observer's Comment (based on general observation):		
	Signature of the Observer		

Introduction: Anatomically speaking, Traube's (semilunar) space has some clinical significance. It is a crescent-shaped area that is bounded by the inferior margin of the left lobe of the liver, the left costal margin, the anterior border of the spleen, and the lower edge of the left lung.

The stomach, which is located beneath Traube's space, causes percussion to make a tympanic sound. Although this can also be a typical finding following a meal, dullness to percussion across Traube's space may indicate splenomegaly. It may also signal other diseases, such as an enlarged left lobe of the liver, a fundus mass, a left pleural effusion, or a significant pericardial effusion. It could be more challenging to evaluate dullness to percussion in obese persons.

Expected from a Student:

1. The student should know about the location of the traube's space.
2. Students should be aware of the normal percussion findings in this region.
3. Students should be well acquainted with the condition in which it is altered.

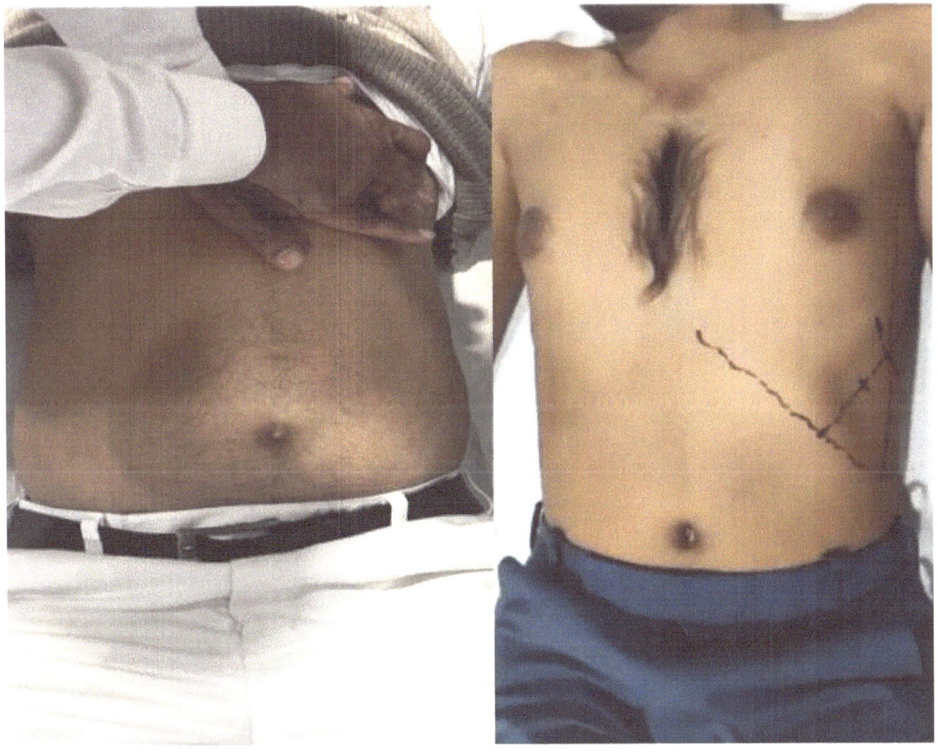

Figure D.1: Demonstrating the method to percuss and outline of traube's area

Clinical application:

- Normal traube's space – Resonant note due to empty stomach.
- Obliteration of Traube'sspace – massive splenomegaly
- Left side pleural effusion
- Pericardial effusion
- Enlarged left lobe of the liver
- Full stomach or fundic mass.

Chapter 4

Gastrointestinal System

A. Palpation of Liver

Table A.1: Checklist

Type of Station: Procedural station

Domain: Cognitive, Psychomotor, Affective.

Communication Time: 1 minute

Marks-10

Sr. no	Steps	Marks	R.no
I	**Checklist**		
1	Stood on the Right side of the patient,madethesubject comfortable in lying down position, and explained the procedure to the patient	1	
2	Exposed the abdomen fully up to the xiphisternum	1	
3	Ensure that his own hands are warm	1	
4	Asked the subject to take a deep breath in and out, both hips flexed	1	
5	Started examination from lower abdominal quadrant from right side with hand keeping parallel to the abdomen	1	
6	Know the dipping method in case of distension of the abdomen	1	
7	Described liver in terms of enlargement (inmidclavicularline), tenderness, its border, surface	2	
II	**Assessment of Professional Behavior**		
1.	Addressed the patient appropriately and introducedhimself/herself by name.	1	
2.	Informed patient regarding completion of the procedure and thanked the patient before leaving	1	
III	**Total Marks (Tick)**	10	
	Final Score		
	Global Rating: 1. Poor; 2. Unsatisfactory; 3. Satisfactory; 4. Good; 5. Excellent		
	Observer's Comment (based on general observation):		
	Signature of the Observer		

Introduction:

Students will be evaluated for palpation of liver by different methods and how to assess liver span. The student needs to understand the clinical technique and interpretation of liver palpation. An enlarged liver may or may not have noticeable symptoms. Causes for an enlarged liver may be evaluated by assessing the surface and consistency of the liver on palpation. Traditionally, the extent of hepatomegaly is expressed in centimeters perceptible below the right costal margin, which should ideally be measured using a ruler. Hepatomegaly can also be described as displacement that is measured in fingerbreadths. Determine the characteristics of the liver surface (i.e. whether it is soft, smooth, and tender as in heart failure, very firm and regular as in obstructive jaundice and cirrhosis, or hard, irregular, painless, and sometimes nodular as in advanced secondary carcinoma).

Expected from a student:

1. The student should be aware of the steps of palpation of the liver
2. The student should be aware of the various methods of liver palpation
3. The student should be able to correlate palpatory findings with symptomatology.
4. The student should be acquainted with the proper steps of the measurement of liver span.
5. Different causes of hepatomegaly and correlate with consistency and the surface of the liver

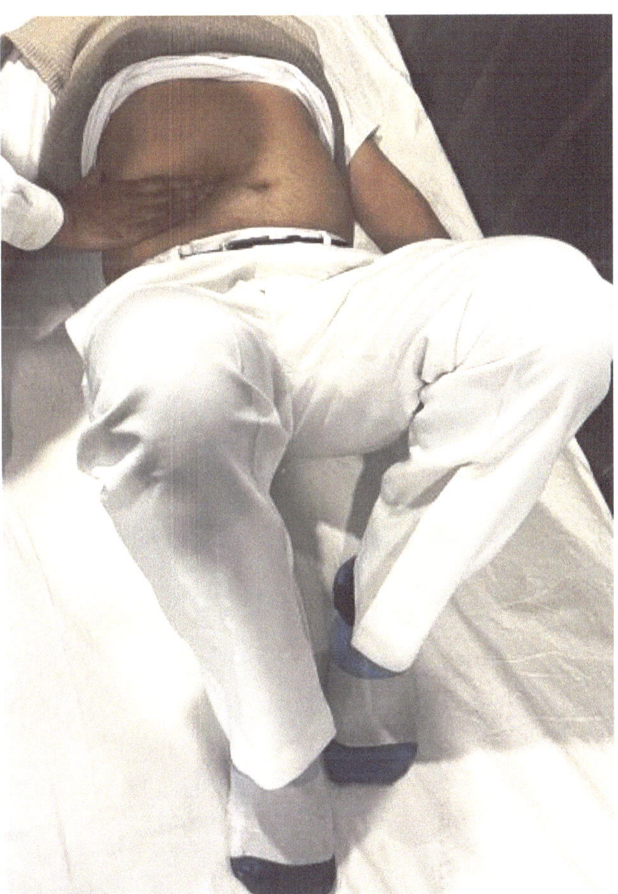

Figure A.1: Demonstrating the method for palpation of the liver

Table A.2: Showing causes of hepatomegaly

INFECTIVE:-	DIGESTIVE AND INFILTRATIVE:-
• Cholangitis • Amoebiasis • Malaria, Kala – azar • Actinomycosis • Histoplasmosis • Echinococcosis **CONGESTIVE:-** • Congestive heart failure/Cardiomyopathy	• Lymphomas • Multiple Myeloma **STORAGE DISORDERS:-** • Niemann – Pick diseases • Gaucher's diseases • Amyloidosis • **Neoplasia** • **Toxins** • Alcohol, Arsenic.

B. Palpation of Spleen

Table B.1: Checklist

Type of Station: Procedural station

Domain: Cognitive, Psychomotor, Affective.

Communication Time: 1 minute

Marks-10

Sr. no	Steps	Marks	R.no
I	**Checklist**		
1	Stood on the Right side of the patient, made the subject comfortable in lying down position, and explained the procedure to the patient	1	
2	Exposed the abdomen fully up to the xiphisternum	1	
3	Ensure that his own hands are warm	1	
4	Asked the subject to take a deep breath in and out, both hips flexed	1	
5	Started examination from right iliac fossa with hand keeping parallel to the abdomen	1	
6	Movement of the palpating finger should go and point towardtheleft upper quadrant of the abdomen	1	
7	Know the dipping method in case of distension of the abdomen	1	
8	Described spleen in terms of enlargement (in midclavicular line), tenderness, its border, surface	1	
II	**Assessment of Professional Behavior**		
1.	Addressed the patient appropriately and introducedhimself/herself by name.	1	
2.	Informed patient regarding completion of the procedure and thanked the patient before leaving	1	
III	**Total Marks (Tick)**	10	
	Final score		
	Global Rating: 1. Poor; 2. Unsatisfactory; 3. Satisfactory; 4. Good; 5. Excellent		
	Observer's Comment (based on general observation):		
	Signature of the Observer		

Introduction: Students should be able to palpate the Spleen by various methods.

Expected from students:

1. The student should know the surface marking of Spleen.
2. The student should know the methods and steps of spleen palpation.
3. The student should know important medical causes of splenomegaly
4. The student should know the salient points of identification of the organ as the spleen.
5. **The student should know the Grading of splenomegaly**
6. The student should know the approach to a case of splenomegaly
7. The student should know the definition and causes of massive splenomegaly

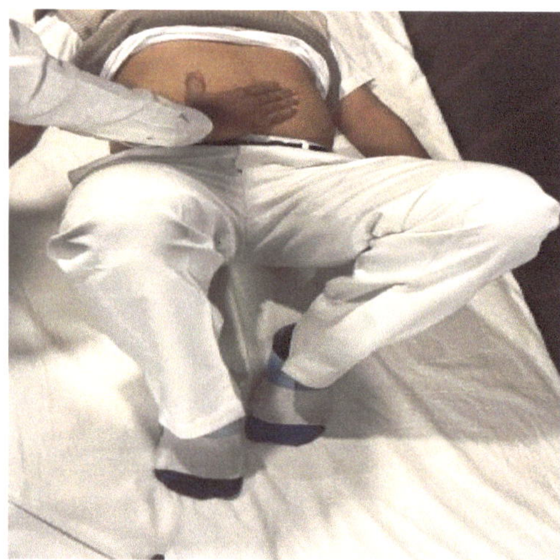

Figure B.1: Demonstrating the palpation of spleen

Introduction: Students should be able to palpate the Spleen by various methods.

Palpation can be accomplished by bimanual palpation and percussion method.

Bimanual palpation: The patient is supine with flexed knees. The examiner's left

hand is placed on the lower rib cage and pulls the skin toward the costal margin, allowing the fingertips of the right hand to feel the tip of the spleen as it descends while the patient inspires slowly. Palpation begins with the right hand in the left lower quadrant with gradual movement toward the left costal margin, thereby identifying the lower edge of anenlarged spleen.

[When the spleen tip is felt, the finding is recorded as centimeters below the left costal margin,10–15 cm, from the midpoint of the umbilicus or the xiphisternal junction].

Percussion method: Splenic dullness demonstrated by Nixon, Castell, or Barkun.

1. Nixon's method: The patient is placed on the right side. Percussion begins at the lower level of pulmonary resonance in the posterior axillary lineand proceeds diagonally along a perpendicular line toward the lower mid-anterior costal margin.

[The upper border of dullness is normally 6–8 cm above the costal margin. Dullness >8 cm in an adult is presumed to indicate splenic enlargement.]

2. Castell's method: With the patient supine, percussion in the lowest intercostal space in the anterior axillary line (eighth or ninth)produces a resonant note if the spleen is normal in size. A dull percussion note in full inspiration suggests splenomegaly.

3. Percussion of Traube'sspace: The borders of Traube'sspace are the sixth rib above, the left midaxillary line laterally,and the left costal margin below. The patient is supine with the left arm slightly abducted. During normal breathing, this space is percussed from medial to lateral margins, yielding a normal resonance sound. A dull percussion note suggests splenomegaly.

Causes of massive splenomegaly:

Myeloproliferative disease, Leishmaniasis, Malaria (tropical splenomegaly syndrome), Portal vein obstruction/portal hypertension, Schistosomiasis, Mucopolysaccharidosis, Lymphomas, Gaucher disease, Hereditary spherocytosis, Thalassemias major.

Causes of mild to moderate splenomegaly:

Bacterial sepsis, Infective endocarditis, Sickle cell disease, Splenic abscess, Acute infectious illnesses (eg, typhoid, malaria), infectious mononucleosis, Systemic lupus erythematosus, Tuberculosis, Banti disease, Immune hemolytic anemias, Immune thrombocytopenic disorders, Symptomatic human immunodeficiency virus infection.

C. Palpation of Kidneys

Table C.1: Checklist

Type of Station: Procedural station

Domain: Cognitive, Psychomotor, Affective.

Communication Time: 1 minute

Marks-10

Sr. no	Steps	Marks	R.no
I	**Checklist**		
1	Stood on the Right side of the patient,made the subject comfortable in lying down position, and explained the procedure to the patient	1	
2	Exposed the abdomen fully up to the xiphisternum	1	
3	Ensure that his own hands are warm	1	
4	Asked the subject to take a deep breath in and out, both hips flexed	1	
5	Started examination by putting a right hand behind the abdomen towards the renal angle	1	
6	Keeping the left hand on the abdomen near the umbilicus, feeling the kidney by pushing from the hand which is behind the abdomen.	1	
7	Looked for the ballotability of the kidney	1	
8	Examined another kidney as well	1	
II	**Assessment of Professional Behavior**		
1.	Addressed the patient appropriately and introducedhimself/herself by name.	1	
2.	Informed patient regarding completion of the procedure and thanked the patient before leaving	1	
III	**Total Marks (Tick)**	10	
	Final Score		
	Global Rating: 1. Poor; 2. Unsatisfactory; 3. Satisfactory; 4. Good; 5. Excellent		
	Observer's Comment (based on general observation):		
	Signature of the Observer		

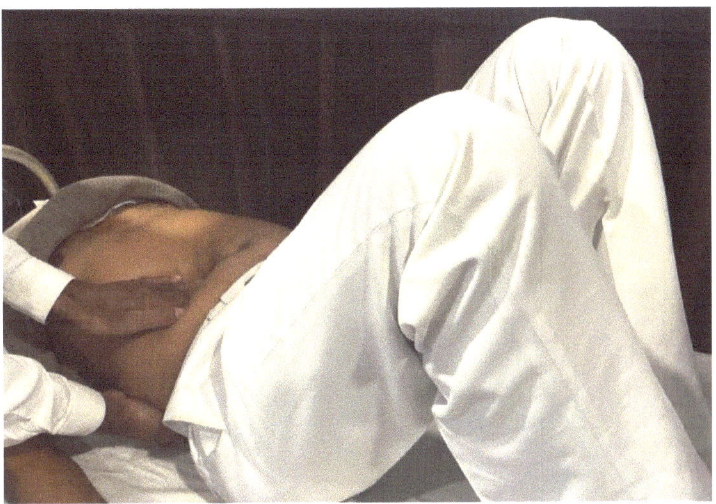

Figure C.1: Demonstrating the method to palpate the kidney

D. Demonstration of Fluid Thrill and Shifting Dullness

Skill station: Fluid Thrill

Table D.1: Checklist
Type of Station: Procedural station
Domain: Cognitive, Psychomotor, Affective.
Communication Time: 1 minute

Marks-10

Sr. no	Steps	Marks	R.no
I	**Checklist**		
1	Stands on the right side of the subject and makesthesubject comfortable in lying down position and explains the procedure.	1	
2	Exposed the abdomen fully up to just above the xiphisternum.	1	
3	Flexes the legs of the patient.	1	
4	Asked the patient to keep the ulnar border of his hand pressed firmly in the midline of the abdomen.	2	
5	Kept left hand on the left side of the abdomen.	1	
6	Flicked the lateral abdominal wall on the right side.	1	
7	Felt the thrill on the left side of the abdominal wall.	1	
II	**Assessment of Professional Behavior**		
1	Addressed the patient appropriately and introducedhimself/herself by name.	1	
2	Informed patient regarding completion of the procedure and thanked the patient before leaving	1	
III	**Total Marks (Tick)**	10	
	Final Score		
	Global Rating: 1. Poor; 2. Unsatisfactory; 3. Satisfactory; 4. Good; 5. Excellent		
	Observer's Comment (based on general observation):		
	Signature of the Observer		

Introduction:

Students will be evaluated for knowing how to interpret the clinical significance of the presence of fluid thrill. Students must know how to evaluate for the presence of free fluid in the abdomen.

Ascites is defined as the accumulation of free fluid in the peritoneal cavity. There are multiple methods to assess the amount of free fluid. The presence of fluid thrill indicates that fluid amounts to more than 2 liters.

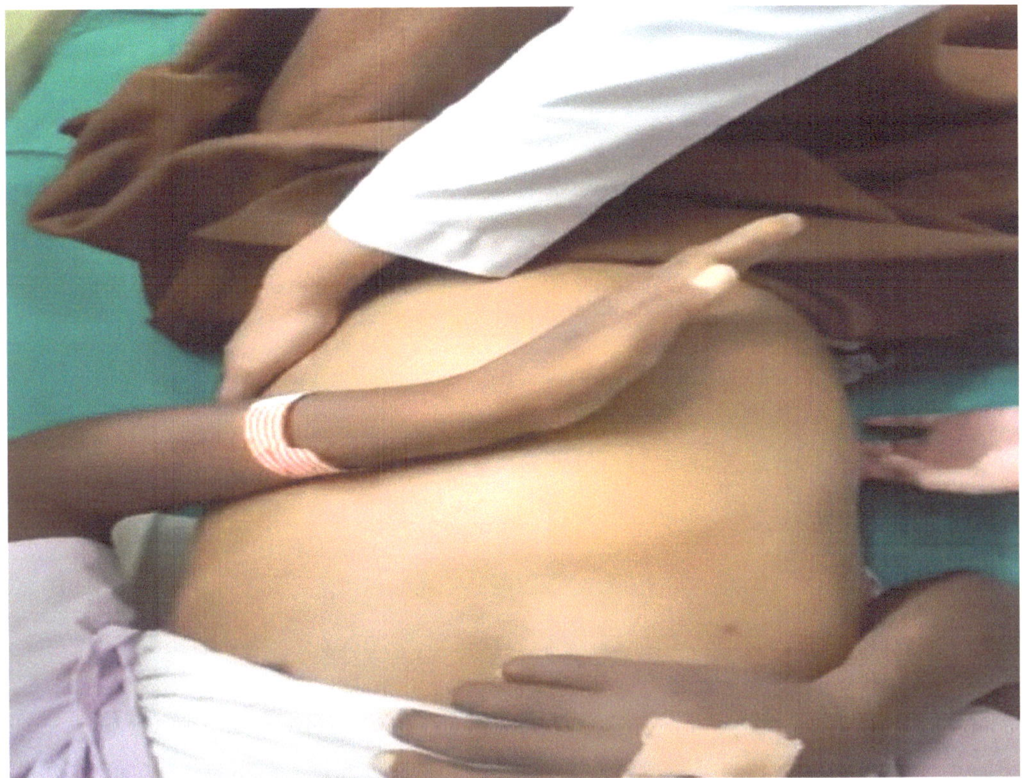

Figure D.1: Demonstrating the method for fluid thrill

Clinical Application:

1. Diagnosis of ascites clinically and to estimate the amount of fluid present
2. Ascertain the cause of ascites

Notes:

SAAG (The cause of ascites can be determined using the serum ascites-albumin gradient marker. A gradient of more than 1.1 g/dl is indicative of portal hypertension in the patient.

Ascites may result from the portal hypertension suggested by **high SAAG** levels. following causes:

- Cirrhosis of the liver, Alcoholic hepatitis
- Portal vein thrombosis
- Budd-Chiari syndrome
- Idiopathic portal fibrosis
- Liver metastasis
- Heart failure, Constrictive pericarditis

Low SAAG causes of ascites:

- Peritoneal carcinomatosis
- Tubercular peritonitis
- Pancreatitis
- Nephrotic syndrome
- Biliary ascites
- Serositis
- Bowel obstruction/infarction

Other methods to demonstrate the presence of free fluid in the abdomen:

- Horseshoe dullness
- Shifting dullness
- Puddle sign

Points to remember:

• The ascites become tense as fluid thrill (fluid more than 2 liters) appears; when fluid levels rise, the mesentery is stretched and bowl loops float in the fluid. The intestinal loops become submerged in more fluid as the mesentery can only stretch so far. At this point, flowing pleasure takes the place of fluctuating dullness. It's known as large ascites.

Skill station: Shifting Dullness

Table D.2: Checklist

Type of Station: Procedural station

Domain: Cognitive, Psychomotor, Affective.

Communication Time: 1 minute   Marks-10

Sr. no	Steps	Marks	R.no
A	**Checklist**		
1	Stands on the right side of the subject and makesthesubject comfortable in lying down position and explains the procedure.	1	
2	Exposes the abdomen of the subject up to the xiphisternum above and pubic symphysis below	1	
3	Flex the knee of the subject	1	
4	Starting from epigastrium percuss in the midline from above downwards till the maximum point of tympanic note	1	
5	From maximum point of tympanicity in midline percuss laterally to one side with pleximeter finger parallel to the long axis of abdomen till you get a dull note	1	
6	Turn the patient to the opposite lateral position and wait for a few seconds (30-60 secs)	1	
7	Percuss again at the same point which will now reveal tympanic resonance	1	
8	Looked for Divarication of recti in ascites by asking the patient to lift the head while giving resistance on the chest.	1	
B	**Assessment of Professional Behavior**		
1	Addressed the patient appropriately and introduced himself/herself by name	1	
2	Informed patient regarding completion of the procedure and thanked the patient before leaving	1	
	Total Marks (Tick)	10	
	Final score		
	Global Rating: 1. Poor; 2. Unsatisfactory; 3. Satisfactory; 4. Good; 5. Excellent		
	Observer's Comment (based on general observation):		
	Signature of the Observer		

Introduction:

Students will be evaluated for demonstration of Shifting dullness. The student needs to understand the clinical technique and interpretation of the shifting dullness. The shifting dullness is a bedside clinical test for the presence of free fluid in the abdomen (ascites).

Expected from a student:

- The student should be acquainted with the proper steps of eliciting shifting dullness.
- The student needs to be aware of the expected result and its interpretation.

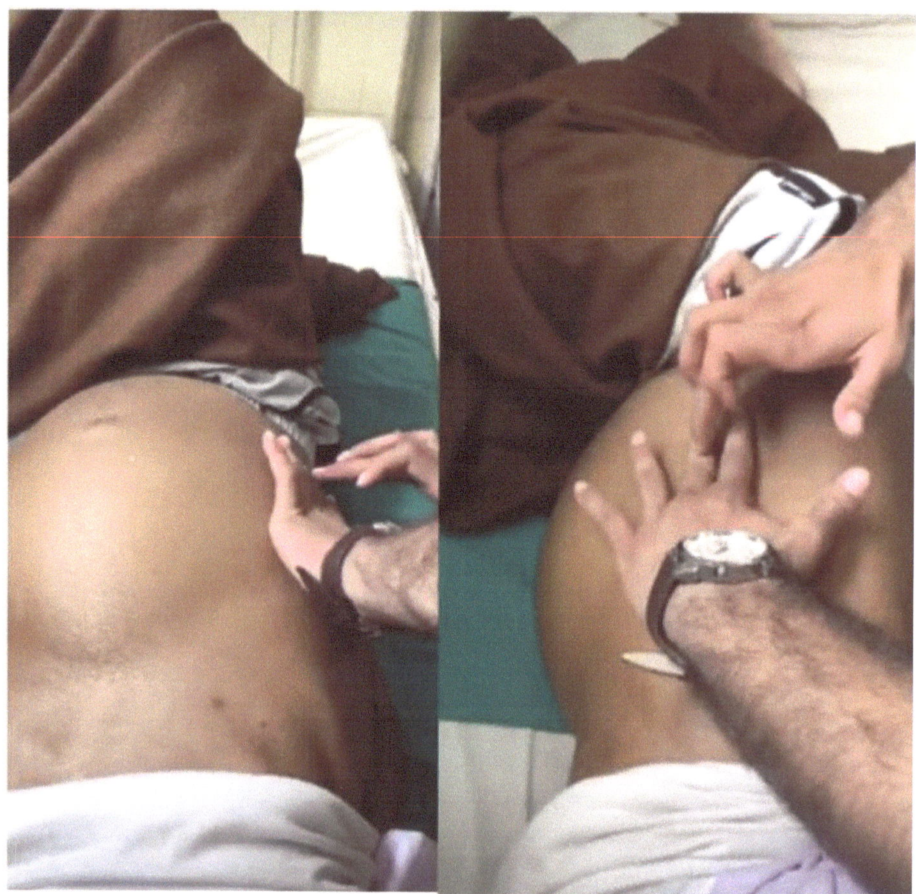

Figure D.2:Demonstrating Shifting dullness

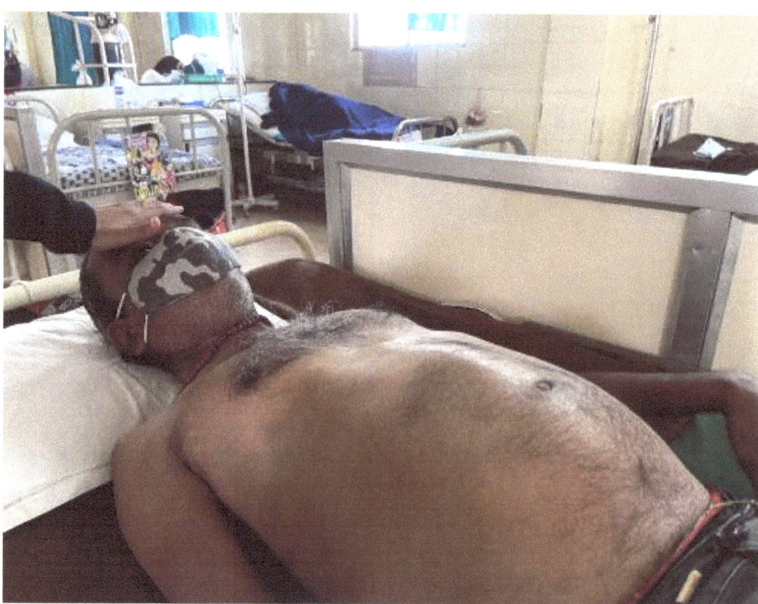

FigureD.3: Demonstration of Divarication of recti in ascites.

Clinical application:

- Eliciting shifting dullness
- Knowledge of bedside signs of ascites
- Causes of ascites

Notes:

Shifting dullness:

By changing the patient's position and displaying a shift in the location of the air-fluid interface, ascites can be validated (i.e., the distinct transition zone between tympany and dullness). It takes at least 1/2 to 1 liter of fluid to show shifting dullness.

Procedure: The intestine floats in the midline while the patient is supine (in healthy persons as well as in ascites). The midline (tympanic) is pounded first, followed by the flanks (dull), following the cardinal rules of percussion, or from a more resonant to a less resonant area. Repeat this after having the patient empty their bladder because the dullness may be caused by a bloated bladder.

Absent shifting dullness: Moving dullness may not be present in loculated ascites, tuberculous peritonitis, tiny collections of free fluid, huge tense ascites, or adherent bowel when there is fluid in the abdomen.

Unilateral shifting dullness: This is known as Balance's sign and is seen in splenic rupture. The blood present in the right side (hemoperitoneum) is pushed to the left side, while the blood present in the left flank becomes clotted (near the spleen) and does not shift to the right side in the right lateral position.

False positive shifting dullness: In paralytic ileus shifting dullness is present but there is no fluid in the abdomen.

Other methods to demonstrate the presence of free fluid in the abdomen:

- Horseshoe dullness
- Fluid thrill
- Puddle sign

Chapter 5

Cardiovascular System

A. Examination of Precordium

Table A.1: Checklist
Type of Station: Procedural station
Domain: Cognitive, Psychomotor, Affective.
Communication Time: 1 minute

Marks-10

Sr. no	Steps	Marks	R.no
I	**Checklist**		
1	Stands on the right side of the subject and makesthesubject comfortable in lying down position and explains the procedure.	1	
2	Exposes the precordium of the patient.	1	
3	Stands at the foot end of the subject to examine for precordial bulge.	1	
4	Identifies the position of apex beat on inspection by observing the patient in supine, left lateral position, and sitting and leaning forward	1	
5	Identifies the position of apex beat by palpation, first identifies with palm and localizes with fingertips. Must look in all the positions for inspection.	1	
6	Examines for left parasternal pulsation or heave using the heel of the palm or ulnar border.	1	
7	Examines for aortic and pulmonary area. Both visible pulsations and palpable heart sounds and murmurs.	1	
8	Examines for sternoclavicular and epigastric pulsations.	1	
II	**Assessment of Professional Behavior**		
1	Addressed the patient appropriately and introduced himself/herself by name	1	
2	Informed patient regarding completion of the procedure and thanked the patient before leaving	1	
III	**Total Marks (Tick)**	10	
	Final Score		
	Global Rating: 1. Poor; 2. Unsatisfactory; 3. Satisfactory; 4. Good; 5. Excellent		
	Observer's Comment (based on general observation):		
	Signature of the Observer		

Introduction:

Students will be evaluated for examination of precordium. The student needs to understand the clinical technique and interpretation of the findings. The examination of the precordium must include inspection and palpation. Inspection must include ruling out any precordial bulge and identifying apex beat. Palpation of precordium should be done using fingertips for identifying pulsations, metacarpal heads for appreciating thrills(palpable murmurs), and the heel of the hand to appreciate any heaves.

Expected from a student:

- The student should be well-oriented with the proper method of examination.
- The student needs to be aware of the expected result and its interpretation.

Clinical application:

- Examination of precordium.
- Identifying apex beat and its character.
- Identifying parasternal heave and its grade.
- Identifying any other pulsations or thrills.

Examination of the Precordium.

The examination of the precordium first includes exposing the precordium. Precordium is that area which is directly overlying the heart. Examination of precordium should be done in the following steps-

1. The first step includes an examination of any precordial bulge; the causes could be – **cardiovascular** – Cardiac enlargement, pericardial effusion

non-cardiovascular causes – skeletal deformity, bronchogenic carcinoma, mediastinalgrowth.

2. **Examination of Apical impulse:** Firstly, we have to observe the position of the apex beat and then confirm the location by palpation, and then comment on its character. If the apical impulse is not visible in the supine position, then the patient should be made to lie in the left lateral position.

3. **Examination of parasternal heave:** It is identified using the heel of the hand over the left sternal margin. The parasternal heave is then graded into 3 grades-

- Grade I – Visible but not palpable
- Grade II – Visible and palpable, but obliterable.
- Grade III – Visible and palpable, but not obliterable.

Parasternal heave could be due to right ventricular enlargement or due to left atrial enlargement. The causes of parasternal heave are-

- **Physiological** – Children, reduced AP diameter.
- **Right ventricular hypertrophy** – Pulmonary stenosis, pulmonary hypertension, TR, VSD, ASD.
- **Left atrial enlargement** – Moderate to severe MS with MR.

4. Examination of aortic and pulmonary pulsations:

Aortic area	Pulmonary area
Visible pulsations- • Aneurysm of aorta • Chronic AR	Visible pulsations- • Pulmonary hypertension • Pulmonary artery dilatation • Pulmonary artery aneurysm
Palpable heart sounds and murmurs-	Palpable heart sounds and murmurs-
• Loud A2 in systemic hypertension • Ejection clicks in the bicuspid aortic valve. • AS • AR with dilated root	• PS – ejection click • Pulmonary hypertension – Diastolic shock. • graham steel murmur

5. Examination of suprasternal pulsations: Suprasternal pulsations are visible in the following conditions-

• Aneurysm of the arch of the aorta
• Aortic dissection
• Aortic regurgitation
• Right aortic arch
• Thyroideaima artery

6. Examination of epigastric pulsations: We examine epigastric pulsations by placing the thumb in the subxiphoid region with a fingertip towards the patient's head, gentle pressure is applied downwards, and the patient is asked to take a deep inspiration. If the impulse is felt on the tip of the fingers, it indicates a right ventricular impulse due to RVH, if the impulse is felt over the pulp of the thumb, it indicates an impulse transmitted from the abdominal aorta (aortic regurgitation or aneurysm of descending abdominal aorta) and if the impulse is felt over the lateral surface of the thumb, it indicates transmitted hepatic pulsations due to TS or TR.

7. Examination of thrills: Thrills are palpable murmurs and are graded from I-IV based on intensity. It is best felt by the metacarpal heads of the hand.

*Continuous thrill in left 1st ICS is due to PDA or rupture of sinus of Valsalva.

* Pericardial knock may be palpable in the mitral area in cases of constrictive pericarditis.

B. Examination of Apex Beat

Table B.1: Checklist

Type of Station: Procedural station
Domain: Cognitive, Psychomotor, Affective.
Communication Time: 1 minute

Marks-10

Sr. no	Steps	Marks	R.no
I	**Checklist**		
1	Stands on the right side of the subject makethesubject comfortable in lying down position and explain the procedure in the local language.	1	
2	Exposes the precordium of the patient.	1	
3	Identifies the position of apex beat on inspection by observing the patient in supine, left lateral position, and sitting and leaning forward	1	
4	Identifies the position of apex beat by palpation, first identifies with palm and localizes with fingertips. Must look in all the positions for inspection.	1	
5	Comment on location, extent, and duration of Apex beat.	2	
6	Comment on abnormalities of the apex	2	
II	**Assessment of Professional Behavior**		
1	Addressed the patient appropriately and introduced himself/herself by name	1	
2	Informed patient regarding completion of the procedure and thanked the patient before leaving	1	
III	**Total Marks (Tick)**	10	
	Final Score		
	Global Rating: 1. Poor; 2. Unsatisfactory; 3. Satisfactory; 4. Good; 5. Excellent		
	Observer's Comment (based on general observation):		
	Signature of the Observer		

Introduction:

Students will be evaluated for the examination of Apex Beat. The student needs to understand the clinical technique and interpretation of the findings. The examination of the Apex beat must include inspection and palpation. Inspection of Apex must include identifying Apex beat. Palpation of Apex beat should be done using the palm and thenlocalized with fingertips.

Expected from a student:

- The student should be well-oriented with the proper method of examination.
- The student needs to be aware of the expected result and its interpretation.

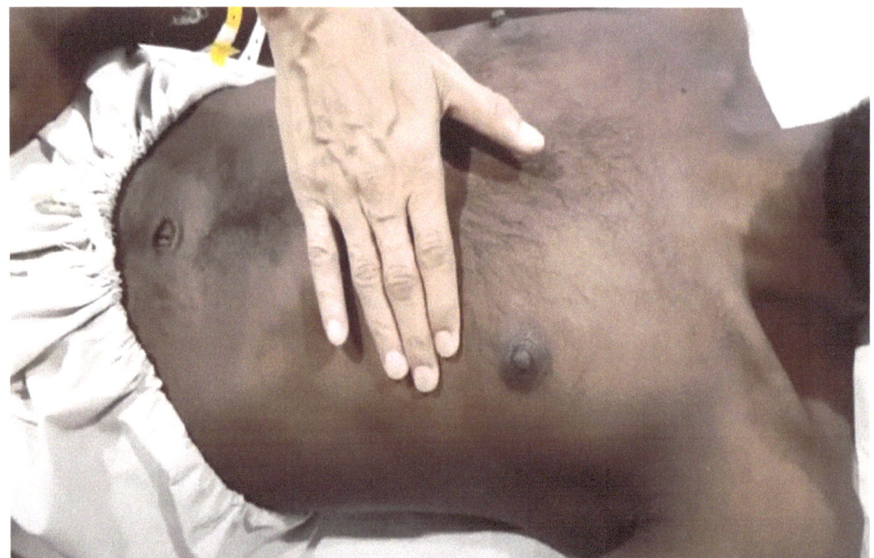

Figure B.1: Demonstrating the method for palpating the apex beat

Clinical application:

- Examination of precordium.
- Identifying apex beat
- Locating apex beat by palpation
- Identifying the character of the apex

Notes:

Examination of the Apex beat: The examination of Apex first includes exposing the precordium. Precordium is that area which is directly overlying the heart. Examination of precordium should be done using a Torch in the following steps-

1. Examination of Apical impulse: Firstly, we have to observe the position of the apex beat and then confirm the location by palpation (first palpate the apex with palm and then localize it with fingertip) and then comment on its character. If the apical impulse is not visible in the supine position, then the patient should be made to lie in the left lateral position.

Features of normal cardiac impulse:

Location – Left 5th ICS, 1–2 cm medial to MCL (or) ≤10 cm from the midsternal line

Extent – <3 cm diameter or one ICS, **Duration** – <50% of systole

2. Mechanism of normal apex: Left ventricular (LV) anterior and anticlockwise rotation brought on by isovolumic contraction during early systole and medial retraction brought on by LV clockwise rotation during late systole.

3. Abnormalities of Apex:

a. Absent (Not seen nor felt) –

- Cardiovascular causes-
    - Pericardial effusion
    - Dextrocardia
- Noncardiac causes-
    - Behind rib
    - Obesity or thick chest wall
    - COPD/emphysema
    - Left-sided pleural effusion
    - Left-sided pneumothorax

b. Tapping – Mitral stenosis (palpable S1-closing snap)

c. Hyperdynamic –

- Increased in amplitude
- Duration is >1/3–<2/3 of systole
- Occupies more than one intercostal space (hence called diffuse apex)

Occurs in LV volume overload conditions:

- Physiological
    - Thin chest
    - Pectusexcavatum
    - High output states
- Pathological
    - AR
    - MR
    - VSD
    - PDA
    - AV fistula

d. Heaving –

- increase in amplitude
- Duration is >2/3 of systole
- Confined to one intercostal space

Occurs in LV pressure overload:

- AS
- Systemic hypertension
- HCM
- Coarctation of aorta

e. Double apical impulse –

- HOCM
- LV aneurysm
- LV dyssynergia

f. Triple or quadruple or wavy impulse – HOCM

g. Retractile – Sever TR

h. See-Saw apex – LV aneurysm

C. Murmurs

Various defects and their corresponding Murmurs are highlighted in the table below as well as figure.

Sr. no	Defects	Murmur
1	Ventricular septal defect (VSD) (Small Muscular VSD/large VSD with pulmonary hypertension	Very Soft (Pin hole/Very large VSD)/Very loud (Moderately Loud VSD) (Maladie de Roger's sign) Early systolic decrescendo murmur of grade I/II/III/IV/V/VI best audible between the apex and left lower sternal border at supine position with the diaphragm of stethoscope in expiration increased on squatting, hand grip or vasopressor agent
2	Atrial septal defect	Ejection systolic murmur inthepulmonary area
3	Patent DuctusArteriosus	Continuous Machinery Murmur in the left second intercostal space (Gibson's area) followed by the first left intercostal space
4	Mitral stenosis	Mid-diastolic,alow-pitched rough rumbling localized murmur of grade I/II/III/IV with pre-systolic accentuation best audible at the mitral area in left lateral position with the bell of the stethoscope in expiration which increases on isometric hand grip.
5	Mitral regurgitation	Soft, high-pitched, Pan systolic Murmur slightly crescendo-decrescendo murmur of grade I/II/III/IV/V/VI best audible at the apex in supine position with the diaphragm of stethoscope radiating to axilla or base of heart accentuated by expiration, squatting, isometric exercise and attenuated by sudden standing, Valsalva, amyl nitrate
6	Mitral prolapse	High-pitched Mid-Late systolic crescendo-decrescendo Murmur best heard at apex radiating to base of heart and axilla (posterior leaflet and anterior leaflet) accentuated by standing, Valsalva
7	Tricuspid stenosis	Mid diastolic Murmur best heard at left lower sternal border with diaphragm of stethoscope increased in inspiration

8	Tricuspid Regurgitation	Pan systolic Murmur heard in the lower left sternal border with the diaphragm of the stethoscope increases in intensity in inspiration (de Carvallo's sign)
9	Aortic stenosis	Ejection systolic crescendo-decrescendo low pitched rough rasping Murmur heard best at base of the heart (right 2nd intercostal space/1st aortic area) in expiration with the diaphragm of stethoscope radiates to both carotids and the apex(Gallavardin's phenomenon)
10	Aortic regurgitation	Soft, high-pitched, early diastolic, decrescendo murmur is usually heard best at the third intercostal space on the left (Erb's point/Neo aortic/second aortic area) with the diaphragm of the stethoscope at the end-expiration with the patient sitting up and leaning forward accentuated in hand grip
11	Pulmonary stenosis	Ejection systolic crescendo-decrescendo murmur best heard inapulmonary area with the diaphragm of the stethoscope which increases in intensity with inspiration
12	Pulmonary regurgitation	High-pitched decrescendo Early diastolic Murmur best heard at left sternal border increased in inspiration
13	Hypertrophic obstructive cardiomyopathy	Mid to late systolic high pitch crescendo-decrescendo murmur just medial to apex accentuated by standing, Valsalva

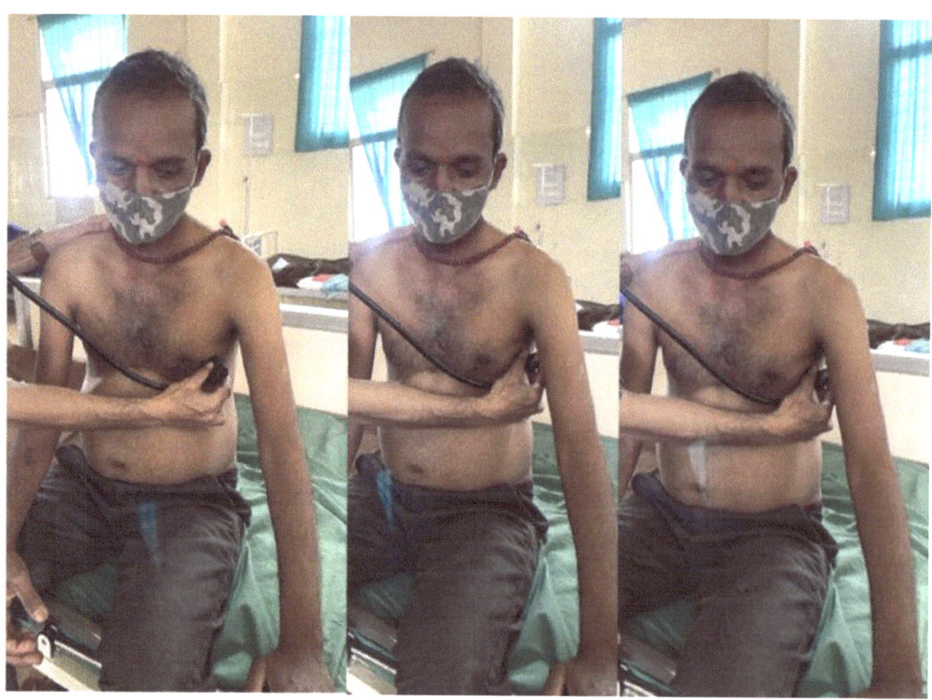

Figure C.1: Demonstration of mitral regurgitation murmur heard best at the apex radiating to the axilla

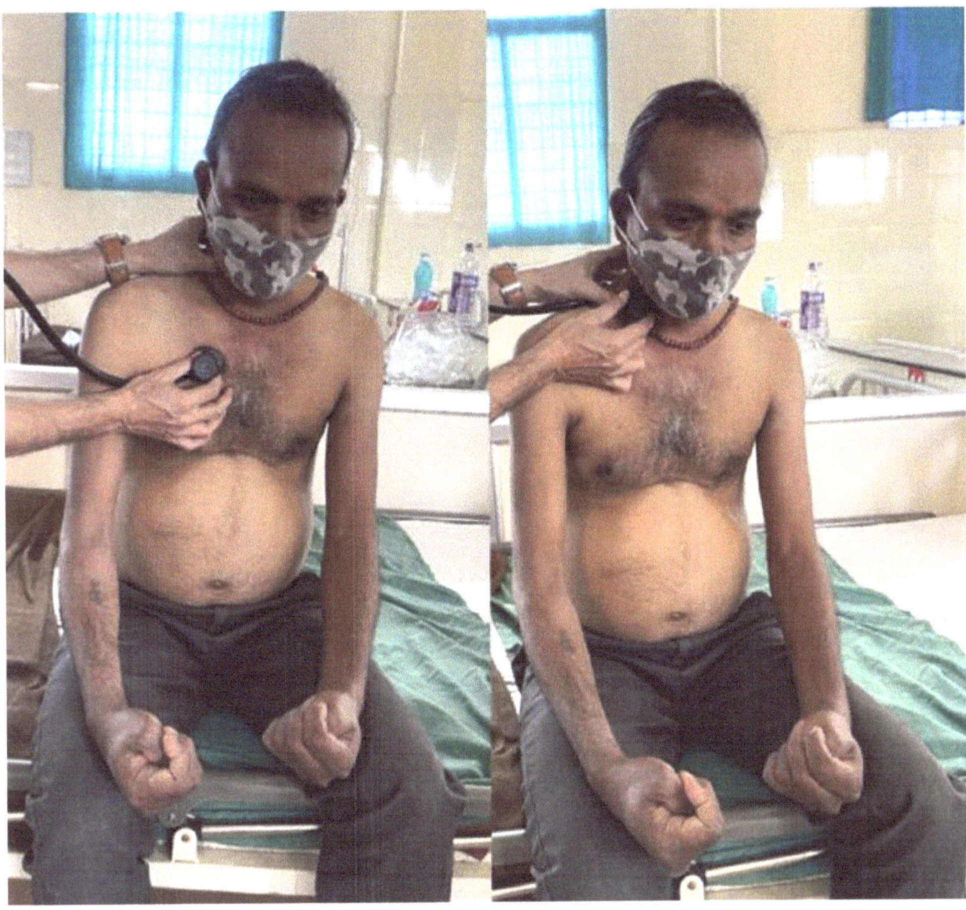

Figure C.2: Demonstration of the murmur of Aortic Stenosis best heard at 1ˢᵗ aortic area radiating to the carotid

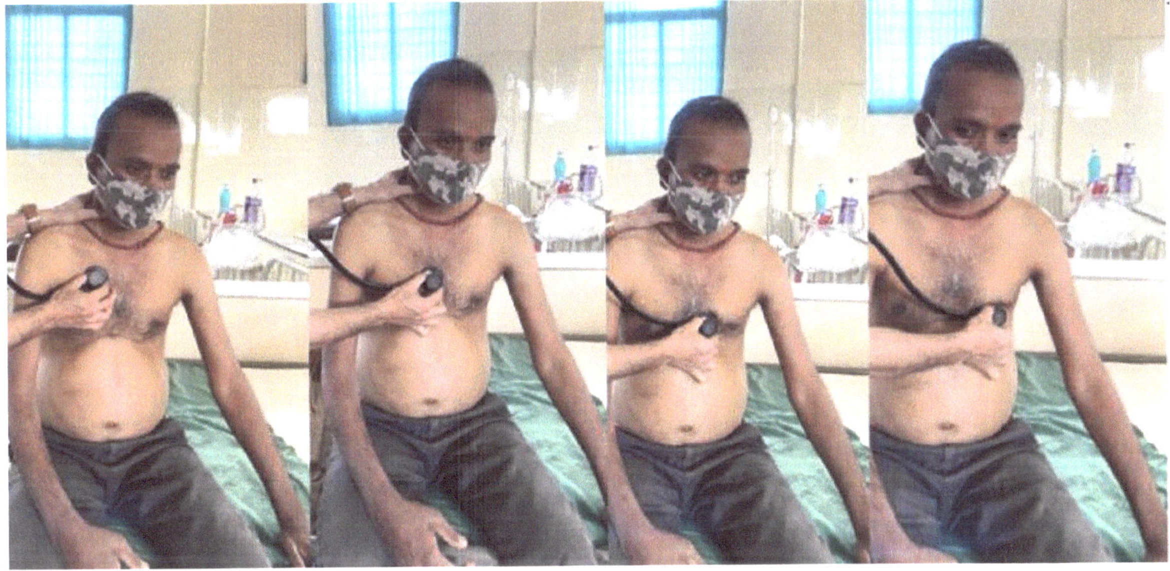

Figure C.3: Aortic stenosis murmur radiating along the aortic Sash area to the apex by inching method
(Gallaverdin Phenomena)

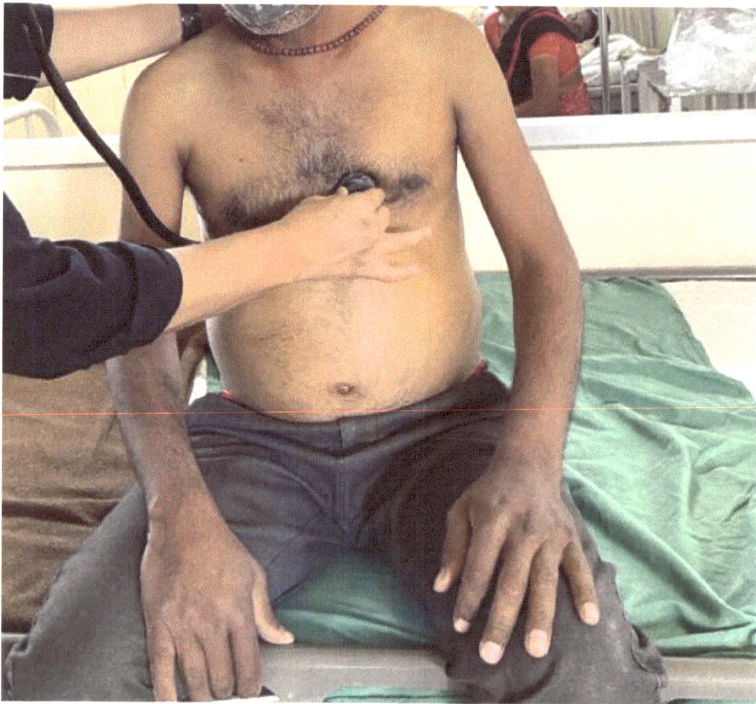

Figure C.4: Demonstration of the murmur of Tricuspid Regurgitation

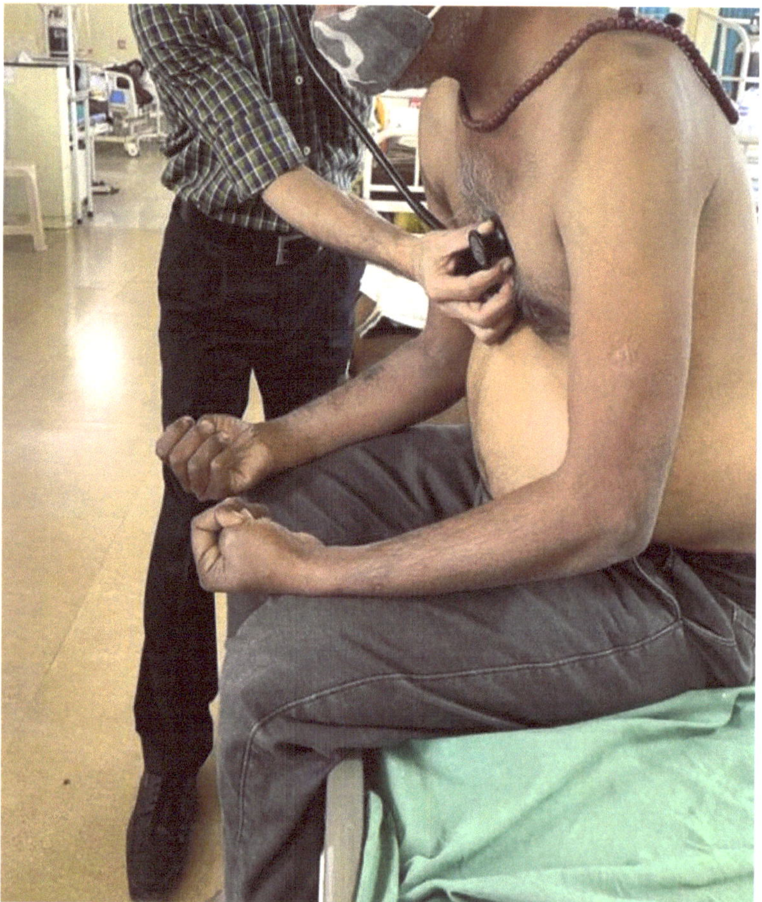

Figure C.5: Demonstration of murmur of Aortic Regurgitation

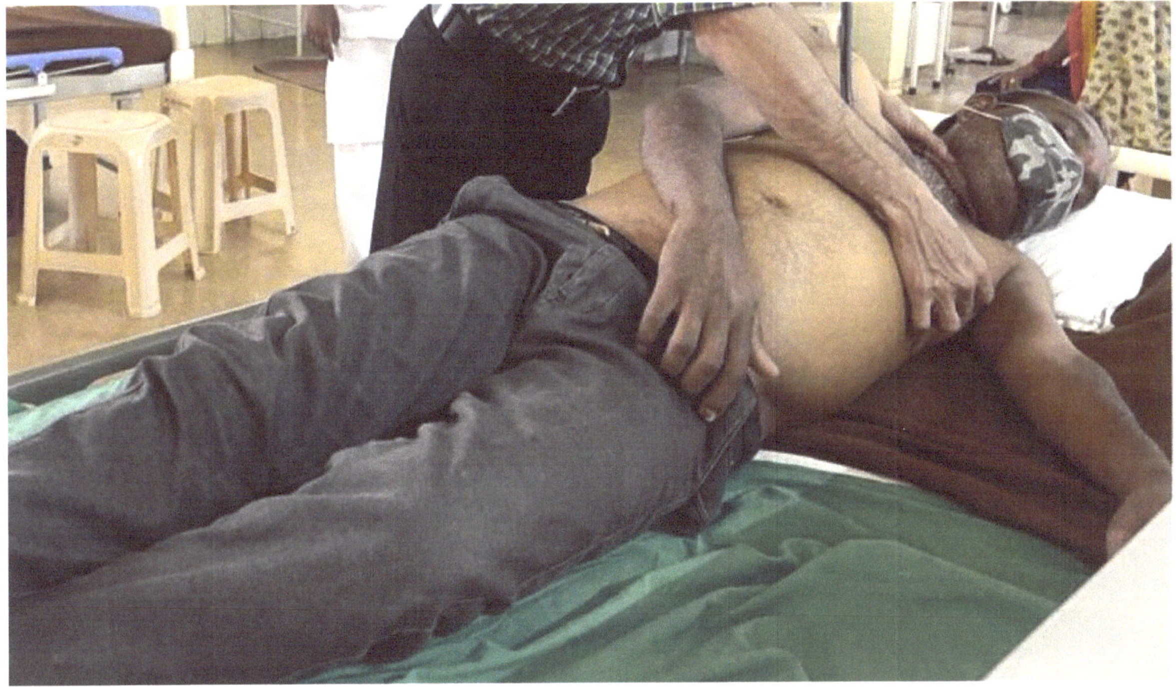

Figure C.6: Demonstration of the murmur of Mitral stenosis best heard in the left lateral position

Chapter 6

OSCE on Attitude, Ethics and Communication (AETCOM)

1. Starting Anti-Seizure Medications

Scenario: A 32-year-old male came with the complains of one episode of generalized tonic-clonic seizure and he must be started on anti-epileptic medication.

Your Task: To convince Patientto start on antiepileptic medication.

Approach to start anti-epileptic medication.

Key issues to explore

- Initially, ascertain the Patient's understanding of his situation. He could be worried that there is nothing that can be done and that the condition is critical, or he can be downplaying how serious the issue is.
- Next, ascertain his knowledge of antiepileptic drugs and his apprehensions regarding their potential adverse effects: Some Patients are worried about long time use of medication whereas others worry about complications.
- Explain why treatment is absolutely needed for his disease.
- Give him informational pamphlets if at all possible, and ask a licensed professional nurse to speak with the Patient if one is present.
- Explain the complications.

Key points to establish

- The Patient need not accept therapy unless he is willing to receive it.
- The informed Patient is free to decline further testing and/or medical intervention.
- Placing the Patient in a situation where they can make well-informed decisions regarding their care is your obligation.

Are they aware of the potential ramifications of the proposed diagnosis?

Appropriate Responses to Likely Questions

Patient: I feel alright.

Student: I understand what you say, you recently experienced a generalized tonic-clonic seizure, and we're here to discuss the initiation of anti-seizure medication.

Patient: However, the condition isn't extremely serious.

Student: I understand that things aren't terrifying right now, but we discovered that you have epilepsy, which might be serious and may worsen. It is possible that treatment can be provided immediately to prevent things from deteriorating further.

Patient: Can you ensure that the issue can be resolved?

Student: No, I am afraid I can't. Until we determine the specific cause.

Patient: I still dislike the thought of taking long-term antiepileptic medications. Is there a viable alternative?

Student: As a matter of fact, there are no other alternatives for your condition.

Patient: Are there any risks or side effects associated with this medication?

Student: That's a valid concern. Like any medication, anti-seizure drugs can have potential side effects. These may include dizziness, drowsiness, changes in mood or behavior, and in some cases, allergic reactions, liver failure in long run. However, it's essential to note that not everyone experiences these side effects, and we carefully monitor Patients for any adverse reactions.

Patient: Will I need to take this medication indefinitely?

Student: The duration of medication will depend on several factors, including your response to treatment, the underlying cause of your seizures, and ongoing assessments. Our aim is to find the right balance where your seizures are well-managed with the least possible medication. If there is a symptom free period for 2 to 5 years then the anti-epileptic medications can be tapered.

Patient: Are there any lifestyle changes or precautions we should be aware of?

Student: Absolutely, maintaining a healthy lifestyle, managing stress, getting adequate sleep, and avoiding triggers can play a significant role in seizure management.

2. Starting Amiodarone Infusion

Scenario: A 74-year-old female had Atrial fibrillation.

Task: To convince Patient relative to start on antiepileptic medication.

Approach to the Patient for Amiodarone infusion.

Key issues to explore

- Inquire about the Patient understanding of their situation. They may be concerned about the severity of their illness or in denial.

- Assess the Patient's knowledge of Atrial Fibrillation and concerns about medication. Patients may be concerned about problems; it's important to put these anxieties in context.
- Explain alternative drugs and the need for amiodarone to provide effective treatment for the Patient's condition.

Key points to establish

- The Patient does not have to consent to any investigation or treatment unless he wants to.

Appropriate responses to likely questions

Patient: I feel alright now.

Student: I understand what you say, however you mentioned that you had chest discomfort and palpitations, so you visited the doctor. Electrocardiogram is showing Atrial Fibrillation.

Patient: Is it a serious problem.

Student: Yes, it a serious condition as it could lead to blood clot in the heart which inturn could cause embolic phenomenon leading to stroke and death. Treatment for this is crucial. Since the illness is curable, the rate of deterioration can be slowed down to allow for improvement without making the condition worse.

Patient: Can you ensure that the issue can be resolved?

Student: No, I'm sorry, but I can't. Until we identify the precise reason.

Patient:Could you provide any other alternative?

Student: Yes,there are other drugs which can be used. But amiodarone would be a better option. We would not suggest it if there were other options.

Patient: Could I die?

Student: No, I'm afraid that I can't tell you for sure. But chances of death after medication is very rare.

Patient: What are the advantages of this treatment, doctor?

Student: Amiodarone is a potent antiarrhythmic medication that can effectively control irregular heartbeats like atrial fibrillation. By restoring a normal heart rate, we aim to alleviate your symptoms such as palpitations, chest pain, and breathlessness, ultimately improving your overall heart function and quality of life.

Patient: Are there any risks associated with this medication?

Student: It's important to note that like any medication, amiodarone does have potential side effects. These may include nausea, dizziness, changes in vision, and in rare cases, more serious effects on the lungs, liver, or thyroid gland. However, we carefully monitor Patients during treatment to minimize these risks and adjust the dosage as needed.

Patient: How long will I need to receive this infusion?

Student: The duration of the amiodarone infusion will depend on how well your heart responds to treatment and how stable your heart rhythm becomes. Our goal is to achieve a stable rhythm and then transition to oral medication to maintain it long-term.

Patient: Are there any lifestyle changes we should consider along with the medication?

Student: Absolutely. A heart-healthy lifestyle, which includes a balanced diet, regular exercise, stress management, and avoiding triggers like excessive caffeine or alcohol, can significantly enhance your heart health and treatment outcomes in addition to medicine.

3. Chronic Kidney Disease

Scenario: A 62-year-old male with hypertension and diabetes mellitus is now diagnosed with chronic kidney disease.

Task: To explain the Patient relative about the new diagnosis.

Key points to explore

- You were diagnosed with chronic renal disease when you were evaluated in the outpatient department.
- After some time to process the information you were previously provided, you would want to talk to the doctor about a few issues you have.
- You are extremely anxious regarding the diagnosis.
- You are worried about how the ailment will turn out and related issues.
- You ask if there are any viable surgical or other therapy alternatives.
- Assist in avoiding problems and a reduction in renal function.
- Dialysis in the near future.
- When this could occur and whether you eventually need a kidney transplant.

Key points to establish

The Patient is not required to participate in any study or therapy unless he gives his consent.

Appropriate responses to likely questions

Patient: I feel alright now.

Student: I understand what you're saying, however you saw the doctor because you were experiencing dyspnea, pedal edema, and decreased urine output. You also have hypertension and Type II diabetes. Now we have identified that you have chronic kidney disease.

Patient: Is it a serious problem.

Student: Yes, it a serious condition as it could lead to build up of nitrogenous waste in the blood and cause complications and death. Treatment for this is crucial. The rate of deterioration can be slowing down without worsening of the disease.

Patient: Can you ensure that the issue can be resolved?

Student: No, this is a definitive diagnosis and requires continuous monitoring and treatment.

Patient: Is there an alternative?

Student: No, unfortunately not. This disease might progress and you will require continuous renal replacement therapy.

Patient: Could I die?

Student: Unfortunately, I'm not sure I can tell you for sure. But chances of death with continuous monitoring and treatment are rare.

4. Lifestyle Modifications of Chronic Kidney Disease

Scenario: A 62-year-old male with hypertension and diabetes mellitus is now diagnosed with chronic kidney disease.

Task: To explain the Patient relative about the lifestyle modifications to be taken in this disease.

Key points to explore

- You were diagnosed with chronic renal disease when you were last seen in the outpatient department.
- After some time to process the information you were previously provided, you would want to talk to the doctor about a few issues you have.
- You are extremely anxious regarding the diagnosis.
- Explain the benefits of lifestyle modifications, its effect on the body.
- Pay more attention to the specific effects of chronic renal disease on his health than on the condition.
- In the case of chronic renal illness, weigh the benefits of changing one's lifestyle against the dangers and unfavorable information concerning damage. Make sure he does not feel pressured and avoid being judgmental.
- Back off if he appears annoyed. Stay positive and friendly.

Key points to establish

The Patient does not have to consent to any investigations or treatment.

Appropriate responses to likely questions

Patient: What are the lifestyle modifications to be done in this disease? Could you please explain and tell me in detail.

Student: I understand your concerns. Firstly, I want to assure you that managing CKD involves several lifestyle modifications. One of the most crucial aspects is your diet. To lessen the burden on your kidneys, it's critical to regulate your consumption of certain minerals like potassium, phosphorus, and salt. Have you already heard of this?

Patient: Yes, I've heard that diet plays a role, but I'm not sure what exactly I should be eating.

Student: Absolutely. Reducing your salt consumption is essential first. This entails staying away from boxed and processed foods and using herbs and spices rather than salt to season your cuisine. It's also crucial to monitor your potassium and phosphorus intake, so I'd recommend limiting foods high in these nutrients like bananas, oranges, dairy products, and whole grains. Would you like more specific guidance on this?

Patient: Yes, please. I want to know what I can and can't eat.

Student: Of course. I'll provide you with a detailed list of foods to include and avoid. Being physically active and keeping a healthy weight can also help control your blood pressure and blood sugar levels, all of which are critical for kidney function. I recommend aiming for at least 30 minutes of moderate exercise most days of the week. Does that sound manageable for you?

Patient: Yes, I think I can incorporate that into my routine.

Student: Great. Lastly, it's crucial to stay hydrated, but since you have CKD, you'll need to monitor your fluid intake closely. We'll discuss your individual fluid needs and ensure you're not overloading your kidneys. Additionally, if you smoke, quitting is incredibly important as smoking can worsen kidney damage. Have you considered quitting?

Patient: Yes, I know I should quit. I'll try my best.

Student: That's excellent to hear. I can provide resources and support to help you quit. Overall, managing CKD involves a combination of dietary changes, physical activity, fluid management, and smoking cessation. I'll provide you with written information summarizing our discussion today.

5. Diabetes Mellitus

Scenario: A 52-year-old male is diagnosed to have Type II Diabetes Mellitus.

Task: To explain the Patient relative about the new diagnosis.

Key points to explore:

- After some time to process the information you were previously provided, you would want to talk to the doctor about a few issues you have.
- You are extremely anxious regarding the diagnosis.
- You're worried about how the illness will turn out. You enquire what are the alternative treatments and Complications of the disease.

Key points to establish

- The Patient is not required to undertake any examination or treatment unless he gives his consent.

Appropriate responses to likely questions

Patient: I am completely fine.

Student: Although I understand what you're saying, you saw the doctor because of decreased urine production, dyspnea, and pedal edema. Additionally, you have Type II diabetes mellitus and hypertension. Now we have identified that you have chronic kidney disease.

Patient: Is it a serious problem.

Student: Yes, it a serious condition as it could lead to build up of nitrogenous waste in the blood and cause complications and death. Treatment for this is crucial. The rate of deterioration can be slowing down without worsening of the disease.

Patient: Can you ensure that the issue can be resolved?

Student: No, this is a definitive diagnosis and requires continuous monitoring and treatment.

Patient: Is there an alternative?

Student: No, unfortunately not. This disease might progress and you will require continuous renal replacement therapy.

Patient: Could I die?

Student: No, I'm sorry, but I can't be certain. But chances of death with continuous monitoring and treatment are rare.

6. Lifestyle Modification in Diabetes Mellitus

Scenario: A 55yearmale who has been diagnosed with diabetes recently is keen on understanding the lifestyle changes necessary to manage his condition effectively.

Task: To explain the Patient relative about the lifestyle modifications to be taken in Diabetes Mellitus.

Key points to explore

- You are required to interact with the Patient and provide appropriate guidance regarding lifestyle modifications for the management of diabetes mellitus.
- Ensure effective communication, empathy, and clarity in your instructions.
- Address the Patient's concerns and encourage active participation in the discussion.
- Assess the Patient's current understanding of diabetes and its management.
- Discuss the importance of lifestyle modifications in diabetes management.
- Provide guidance on dietary changes, including meal planning, portion control, and carbohydrate monitoring.

- Educate the Patient on the significance of regular physical activity and exercise in diabetes control.
- Address any questions or concerns the Patient may have regarding lifestyle modifications

Key points to establish

The Patient does not have to consent to any examination or treatment unless he is willing to do so.

Appropriate responses to likely questions

Patient: I'm just worried about how I can manage this condition.

Student: I understand. It's completely normal to feel concerned, but there are many lifestyle changes that can positively impact your diabetes management. Let's start with your diet. Have you made any changes to your eating habits since your diagnosis?

Patient: Not really, but I know I need to watch what I eat.

Student: That's a great starting point. A nutritious and healthy diet is essential for diabetic management. Diet rich in vegetables, lean proteins, and whole grains should be included. Try to limit your intake of processed foods, sugary drinks, and high-fat foods. Do you have any dietary requirements or preferences that we should take into account?

Patient: I adore sweets, but I'm not on any particular diet.

Student: Many people enjoy sweets, but it's important to consume them in moderation. Instead of sugary snacks, try incorporating healthier alternatives like fresh fruits or sugar-free options.

Patient: What exercise to be done for my condition?

Student: Regular exercise is another essential component of diabetes management. Every day, try to get in at least 30 minutes of moderate-intensity activity, such brisk walking or cycling. Including two or three weight training sessions a week can also assist to increase insulin sensitivity. Have you been engaging in any regular physical activity?

Patient: I used to go for walks occasionally, but I haven't been very active lately.

Student: That's understandable, but it's never too late to start. Begin by incorporating small changes into your routine, such as taking short walks after meals or finding activities that you enjoy. As your level of fitness rises, gradually increase the length and intensity of your exercises. It's critical to give other areas of self-care, such as controlling stress, getting adequate sleep, abstaining from smoking, and consuming moderation in alcohol, equal priority with nutrition and exercise.

7. Consent for Lumbar Puncture

Scenario: A 42-year-old male presented to medicine department who is a case of suspected meningitis and lumber puncture of the Patient is adviced.

Task: To ascertain the Patient's concerns and convey the rationale behind the additional investigation.

Key issues to explore –

- Inquire about the Patient's understanding of their situation. They may be concerned about the severity of their illness or in denial.
- Assess the Patient's knowledge about Lumbar Puncture and his concern about the procedure.
- Give him informational pamphlets if they are accessible, and ask the specialized nurse to talk with the Patient if one is there.

Key points to establish

- Unless he consents, the Patient is not required to participate in any investigations.
- The Patient will still receive treatment even if he doesn't go through the suggested examinations, but a thorough investigation might enhance the care he receives and help to relieve some of his problems.

Appropriate responses to likely questions

Patient: I'm absolutely fine now.

Student: I can understand, but you have come to the hospital because you have a fever, headache, photophobia, and clinical signs of meningeal irritation and it looks as though this is due to an infection of layers of your brain.

Patient: However, the issue isn't too serious right.

Student: I am aware that the situation is not dire right now, but we have discovered a very dangerous and perhaps worsening brain layer issue. Since the sickness is curable, it's possible that therapy today will make things better so they don't grow worse or that it will slow down the rate of deterioration so that you get better without making the condition worse.

Patient: Can you ensure that the issue can be resolved??

Student: No, I'm afraid I'm not able to. We will be unable to tell you the precise organism that caused this illness until we get that information.

Patient: The thought of having a lumbar puncture still bothers me. Is there a substitute?

Student: Indeed, we will be able to obtain some information from brain scans, which we can perform. Still, the most crucial information that lumbar puncture provides is information that we cannot obtain from any other source, such as the meningitis causing bacterium. If better options were available, we wouldn't advise this.

Patient: Is the procedure painful?

Student: The procedure may cause somediscomfort. The procedure is done in about 10 minutes.

8. Blood Transfusion

Scenario-A 45 year old male present to medicine department who is a case of severe iron deficiency anemia with hemoglobin 5 gm%. Blood transfusion is adviced to the Patient.

Task: To ascertain the Patient's worries and explain the rationale for the blood transfusion

Key issues to explore

- Firstly, the Patienthas to be aware of his condition
- Next, include his knowledge of blood transfusions and his concerns regarding them. While some Patients may be concerned about bad responses to blood transfusions, others may be concerned about the illness being spread through blood transfusions.
- Inform him of any other treatment options that may be available for his disease and the reason for the necessity of a blood transfusion for its management.

Key points to establish

- Patient has the right to deny any treatment or investigation unless consents to it.
- Even if he does not receive the suggested therapy, he will still receive care.

Appropriate responses to likely questions

Patient: I'm feeling absolutely fine.

Student: I know, but you have generalized weakness, black-colored stools, and clinical signs of Iron deficiency anemia and it looks as though this is due to a deficiency of Iron in your body which is the cause of decreased hemoglobin in your blood.

Patient: Yet, the issue isn't that serious.

Student: While things may not be too bad right now, we have discovered a potentially dangerous and perhaps worsening issue with your hemoglobin concentration in the blood. Given that the condition is curable, it's possible that therapy will either make things.

Patient: I still don't like the idea of blood transfusion. Is there an alternative?

Student: Yes, we can and will intravenous injections of ferrous sucrose or ferrous carboxy maltose that increase hemoglobin in your blood to some extent. However, Blood transfusion will cause a definite increase in the amount of hemoglobin in your blood quickly and you will get early relief from the symptoms. We wouldn't recommend this if there were better alternatives.

Patient: Will it lead to any complications?

Student: The blood transfusion carries the risk of several adverse reactions but those are manageable with prompt treatment. We will do it under supervision and monitor vitals also during the transfusion and will stop blood transfusion and give immediate treatment when we suspect adverse reactions. Although only 3 or 4 people out of every 100 people suffer from adverse reactions during blood transfusion and 96 to 97 people undergo blood transfusion without any adverse events.

9. Colonoscopy

Scenario: A 78-year-old male came to the medicine OPD who is a case of bleeding from rectum.

Task: To ascertain the Patient's concerns and convey the rationale behind the additional investigation.

Key issues to explore

- First, identify if the Patient knows about his condition.He can be in denial about how bad the situation is or worried that nothing can be done because he is extremely sick.
- Next, ascertain his knowledge about colonoscopy and any concerns he may have: While some Patients are concerned about discomfort and agony.

Key points to establish

- The Patient does not have to consent to any examination or treatment unless he is willing.
- Even if he chooses not to pursue the recommended investigations, he will still get treatment; nonetheless, a thorough investigation might enhance the care he receives and help to relieve some of his problems.

Appropriate responses to likely questions

Patient: I am fine now.

Student: I can understand it, but you are here because you have abdominal pain, weight loss, loss of appetite, and Laboratory investigations of Gastrointestinal malignancy and it looks as though this is due to a tumor in your gastrointestinal system which has high chances of being malignant.

Patient: The thought of having a colonoscopy bothers me. Can you provide any other substitute?

Student: Yes, we are able to and will perform abdominal scans that will provide us with some data. Nonetheless, the most crucial information is provided by a colonoscopy, since it allows us to get a sample from the lesion—something that cannot be obtained in any other way—and immediately observe any problematic lesions that may be present. In the event that there were better options, we wouldn't advise this.

Patient: Will the procedure be painful?

Student: The procedure can cause some amount of discomfort while it lasts for very short duration. Also, we give local anesthesia before the procedure. This lasts for 15 to 20 minutes and after this, it should not be uncomfortable.

10. Upper Gastro Intestinal Endoscopy

Scenario: A 38 year male who is chronic alcoholic came to medicine department with 3 episodes of hematemesis and large esophageal varices is suspected. He is advised for upper gastrointestinal endoscopy.

Task: To ascertain the Patient's concerns and convey the rationale behind the additional investigation.

Key issues to explore

- First, identify if the Patient knows about his condition. He can be in denial about how bad the situation is or worried that nothing can be done because he is extremely sick.
- Next, ascertain his knowledge about endoscopy and any concerns he may have: While some Patients are concerned about discomfort and agony.

Key points to establish

- The Patient does not have to consent to any examination or treatment unless he is willing.
- Even if he chooses not to pursue the recommended investigations, he will still get treatment; nonetheless, a thorough investigation might enhance the care he receives and help to relieve some of his problems.

Appropriate responses to likely questions

Patient: I am fine now.

Student: I can understand you are feeling better, but you have come to the hospital because you have blood in vomitus almost 3 episodes and you are chronic alcoholic. This looks like you have alcoholic liver disease with portal hypertension causing esophageal varices and treatment of that needs to be done.

Patient: But the problem isn't very bad.

Student: I know you feel this due to all the medications you have been given. However, we believe there may be a major issue with the bleeding blood vessels in your esophagus, which is a part of your upper gastrointestinal tract and might develop worse. Since this is curable, it's possible that therapy today will make things better so they don't grow worse or that it will slow down the rate of deterioration so that you get better without making the condition worse.

Patient: The idea of an upper gastrointestinal endoscopy still bothers me. Is there another option?

Student: Yes, we can get an Abdominal scan that can give us some information. The most crucial information, however, is provided by upper gastrointestinal endoscopy, which allows us to obtain a sample from the lesion if necessary and immediately observe any pathological lesions that may be present. If there were better options, we wouldn't suggest this.

Patient: Is the procedure painful?

Student: Although the treatment is brief, it may cause discomfort during that time. Also, we give local anesthesia before the procedure. This lasts for 15 to 20 minutes and after this, it should not be uncomfortable.

11. Starting Insulin Therapy and Diet Control

Case Scenario:

A 58-year female, who has Type II diabetes mellitus and on oral anti hypoglycemic agents and uncontrolled diet. Her hba1c is 11. She is not keen on taking insulin

Task:

To discuss and explain the need of better control and recommend to start her on insulin therapy.

Key issues to explore

- First identify what the Patient knows about his illness: he may be concerned that the condition is critically ill and nothing can be done or be in denial about the seriousness of the problem.
- Next, ascertain his knowledge of insulin therapy and his concerns over it. While some Patients are concerned about pain and discomfort, others are concerned about complications.
- Explain why insulin is needed to give him.

Key points to establish

- The Patient does not have to consent to any examination or treatment if he doesn't want to.
- Even if he does not take the prescribed insulin, he will still receive treatment; nonetheless, insulin may enhance the care he receives and therefore lessen some of his symptoms.

Appropriate responses to likely questions

Patient: There must be another solution without having to go on insulin.

Student: I understand your concerns about insulin treatment. While insulin is a commonly prescribed medication for diabetes management, there are alternative treatments and strategies available. Let's discuss them together and find the best approach for your individual needs and preferences.

Patient: What type of diet should I take?

Student: A balanced diet is essential for managing diabetes. Focus on incorporating more fruits, vegetables, whole grains, lean proteins, and healthy fats into your meals. Limiting sugary and processed foods can also help control blood sugar levels.

Patient: I'm terrified of needles – can you give me the insulin in any other form?

Student: I understand your fear of needles. There are alternatives to traditional insulin injections, such as insulin pens or pumps, which may be more comfortable for you.

12. Lifestyle Modification Post Myocardial Infarction

Case Scenario:

A 55 year old male Patient who recently got Coronary Angiography done suggestive of double vessel disease and Patient underwent Coronary Angioplasty. Currently he is doing fine and is planned for discharge and is keen on understanding the lifestyle changes necessary to manage his condition effectively.

Task: To explain the Patient relative about the lifestyle modifications to be taken post Myocardial Infarction.

Key points to explore

- You are required to interact with the Patient and provide appropriate guidance regarding lifestyle modifications post MI.
- Address the Patient's concerns and encourage active participation in the discussion.
- Assess the Patient's current understanding of myocardial infarction and its management.
- Discuss the importance of lifestyle modifications post MI

Key points to establish

- The Patient does not have to consent to any inquiry or treatment unless he is willing to do.

Patient: Did I really have a heart attack?

Student: I understand your concern. Based on the tests and results we've reviewed; it appears that you did experience a heart attack. However, we're here to support you through your recovery and help you understand your condition better.

Patient: Did the procedure performed when I arrived at the hospital completely resolve the issue?

Student: The procedure you underwent was a crucial step in addressing the issue. While it may have resolved a part of the problem, we need to continue monitoring your condition and make further recommendations to ensure your long-term health.

Patient: What actions should I take now to prevent future problems?

Student: Moving forward, it's important to focus on lifestyle changes such as maintaining a healthy diet, regular exercise, managing stress, and taking prescribed medications as directed. We'll work together to create a personalized plan to reduce the risk of future issues.

Patient: I'm worried about what to do if a similar situation occurs again. Will the hospital continue to monitor me?

Student: We understand your concerns, and rest assured, we have systems in place for ongoing monitoring and support. We'll schedule follow-up appointments to check your progress, address any new concerns, and ensure you have the necessary resources to manage any future situations effectively.

13. Hypertension

Scenario: A 54-year female has been diagnosed with hypertension and is very anxious about her treatment.

Task: To explain the Patient about the new diagnosis and the treatment modalities for the same.

Key issues to explore

- First, find out what the Patient knows about his condition: he may be concerned that the condition is critically ill and nothing can be done or be in denial about the seriousness of the problem.
- Then establish what he knows about hypertension and his fears about hypertension.

Key points to establish

- Patient does not have to undergo any investigation or treatment unless he agrees to it.

Patient: Doctor, it seems I have hypertension. I'm a bit overwhelmed and not sure what this means for me.

Student: I understand this news can be concerning, but please know that we're here to support you every step of the way. It's important to address hypertension early to manage it effectively and improve your overall health.

Patient: Can you explain what hypertension is and why it's important to manage it?

Student: Hypertension, or high blood pressure, is a condition where the force of blood against your artery walls is consistently high. Managing it is crucial because uncontrolled hypertension can lead to heart disease, stroke, and other serious health issues.

Patient: What can I do to manage my blood pressure?

Student: Lifestyle changes play a key role. We'll focus on dietary modifications, exercise, stress management, and possibly medication, depending on your specific situation. Let's start by discussing dietary modifications.

Patient: I'm worried about taking medication. Are there alternatives?

Student: Medication is one option, but we'll explore non-pharmacological approaches first. Lifestyle changes alone can often make a significant impact on blood pressure. We'll monitor your progress closely and adjust the plan as needed.

Patient: How long will it take to see improvements in my blood pressure?

Student: It varies from person to person, but with consistent efforts and follow-up, we aim to see improvements within a few weeks to months. Regular check-ups will help us track your progress and make any necessary adjustments.

14. Dietary Modification of Hypertension

Scenario: A 62 years old male Patient known case of hypertension for 3 years planned for discharge is keen on understanding the lifestyle changes necessary to manage his condition effectively

Task: To explain the Patient relative about the lifestyle modifications to be taken for hypertension

Key points to explore

- You are required to interact with the Patient and provide appropriate guidance regarding lifestyle modifications for hypertension
- Assess the Patient's current understanding of hypertension and its management.
- Discuss and provide guidance on dietary changes, including meal planning, portion control, and carbohydrate monitoring.
- Educate the Patient on the significance of regular physical activity and exercise in hypertension.

Key points to establish

- Patient does not have to undergo any investigation or treatment unless he agrees to it.

Patient: What specific changes should I make to my diet?

Student: Firstly, focus on reducing your sodium intake. This means cutting back on processed foods, salty snacks, and adding less salt during cooking.

Patient: That makes sense. What about potassium?

Student: Great question! Increasing potassium-rich foods like bananas, oranges, spinach, and sweet potatoes can help balance your sodium levels and lower blood pressure.

Patient: Is there a specific diet plan I should follow?

Student: Yes, the DASH diet (Dietary Approaches to Stop Hypertension) is highly recommended. It emphasizes fruits, vegetables, whole grains, lean proteins, and low-fat dairy products.

Patient: Will I have to give up all my favorite foods?

Student: Not necessarily. You can still enjoy flavorful meals by using herbs, spices, and healthy cooking methods instead of salt. It's about moderation and making healthier choices overall.

Patient: I've heard about lifestyle changes like exercise and stress management. How do they tie into dietary modifications?

Student: Exercise, stress management, and maintaining a healthy weight are all part of a comprehensive approach to managing hypertension. They work synergistically with dietary changes to improve overall health.

www.ingramcontent.com/pod-product-compliance
Lightning Source LLC
Chambersburg PA
CBHW040321140726